Mastering
Sustainable Health

Living In Harmony With The Physical Body

FRAVARTI

Order this book online at www.trafford.com
or email orders@trafford.com

Order this book online at www.fravarti.com

Most Trafford titles are also available at major online book retailers.

Print information available on the last page.

ISBN: 978-1-4907-8318-5 (sc)
ISBN: 978-1-4907-8317-8 (e)

Library of Congress Control Number: 2017909521

Trafford rev. 06/27/2018

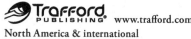 www.trafford.com
North America & international
toll-free: 1 888 232 4444 (USA & Canada)
fax: 812 355 4082

CONTENTS

ACKNOWLEDGEMENT

For the creation of this book I'd like to thank my clients - the thousands of men, women and children who have shared with me some of their darkest hours and greatest challenges. It is one of the greatest privileges of my life to have been included so intimately in the lives of those who have relied on me to provide guidance and support through life's most difficult passages from birth to death. Grief, loss and suffering strips us of our defenses and forces us to be real and to be present to the demands of the realities of our challenges. Being real in this life of illusions and pretensions mostly happens in time of crisis of great magnitude. I learned what I have put in this book through the great courage and striving of people who set goals for themselves and their lives and then set about doing what it would take to create those outcomes and ideals. The path of healing is rigorous and demanding. The rainbow of satisfaction at the end of the journey is the amazing success stories of those who do what it takes, who commit themselves, again and again, if necessary, and seemingly do the impossible because that's what life requires of us.

Additional Acknowledgements:

My gratitude and appreciation to all of these people who helped in the creation of this book.

Eileen Palma - Typing and proof reading
Judy McClellan - Proof reading, and editing
Cyndy Clapp - Proof reading, editing and article: Experiences in Becoming A Medical Intuitive pages 204 - 205
Annette Crotti - Proof reading and resource pages 216 -217 and article: The Joys of Raising Our Severely Allergic Child pages 112 -114
Beret Isaacson - Proof reading and article: Essential Oils for Sustainable Health pages 170 -172
Karen Menke - Proof reading and for rescuing me when I was broken in body and spirit and bereft of any motive to live. Without this help, my life and work would have ended.
Sharia Des Jardins - Cover Photo, layout and design
Annette Stoesser, M.D. -for teaching me about intravenous therapies

Patch Adams, M.D. - for teaching me that happiness creates health

Pir Vilayat Inayat Khan - for training in spiritual practice and intuition

Ellen Silverman, R.N. - for suggesting the 12 week protocol

Marguerite Sears - for corrections, final editing, layout and design including cover. My friendship with Marguerite has strengthened my faith and profoundly influenced my personal experience of God through the message of the prophet Baha'u'llah

INTRODUCTION

Health is a journey towards a moving target. As we make changes to our life with the purpose of improving our health and the layers of disease peel away, new paths are revealed directing us to the next step in our journey. Fravarti is an expert guide to have along the way. Her years of experience, dedication to holistic healing and living, and passion for continuing to grow personally make her an excellent consultant for your journey to health and healing. Her ability to read the signposts on the journey that are pointing us in the direction of whole health and permanent cure are amazingly accurate. This book is her road map for the journey to optimal health and living.

Fravarti has assisted and supported thousands of clients in their personal healing of a wide range of maladies and diseases ranging from the common cold to cancer; low-grade depression to chronic PTSD and more. Many of these people were without hope since no cure could be found in traditional medicine. Fravarti passionately believes in the body's innate ability and desire to heal itself, if we will only listen and follow the direction that is revealed.

Fravarti's first book, *Mastering Homeopathy: The Art of Permanent Cure*, explains the use of homeopathic remedies in the pursuit of health and healing. In this book, *Mastering Sustainable Health*, Fravarti offers a comprehensive guide to overall lifestyle, health care, and maintenance for optimal living. She addresses all body levels: physical, mental, emotional, spiritual, and moral (how we relate to others in the world), which are equally important to address while working towards improved health and well-being.

Her approach is unconventional in that it works from a health-centered model rather than the disease centered model of conventional western medicine. There has been an increase in the merging of these two approaches as traditional medical professionals are beginning to utilize alternative approaches to healing rather than merely treating symptoms. Based on her belief that the body has the desire and power to heal, Fravarti goes to the root of the problem seeking permanent cure rather than only treating symptoms for comfort and relief. While considered unconventional by some, still hundreds of traditional medical professionals consult her for her wisdom and expertise with their own patients.

Fravarti's journey began in 1974 with the home birth of her second child while deeply involved with a community in Fairfax, Virginia, started by Dr. Patch Adams, M.D. The community was comprised of many traditionally trained medical professionals and alternative healers, all pursuing information and experience with the healing properties of alternative modalities. Having suffered with poor health since childhood, Fravarti passionately embraced the healing modalities she experienced during her time in this community for herself and her children, who were also born with health challenges. Inspired by her experiences, Fravarti came to believe that true healing was possible for anyone.

In 1978, Fravarti took her next step becoming formally trained as a midwife in Tucson, Arizona while continuing her study of natural healing alternatives. In 1989, Fravarti was hired to manage the supplement department of a health food store in Charlotte, NC. This provided the perfect setting for the next essential piece of her education. She quickly learned about these supplements, began to informally consult with people and assist them in discovering alternative solutions to their health issues. Customers would frequently stand in line to avail themselves of her experience and support. It soon became apparent that she had discovered her calling and it was time to establish her own consulting practice. Since 1993, Fravarti has been working as a dedicated intuitive health consultant.

When Fravarti works with her clients, she is always speaking in terms of the ideal. She honors and recognizes the commitment many of these changes will require. She does not mince words in terms of what is truly needed, while simultaneously bringing a compassionate eye of understanding for what this path requires. Fravarti is aware that making pervasive lifestyle changes can seem impossibly hard and daunting at the start, and she also knows that once the journey has begun, it is not as hard as it seemed. Her compassion and understanding is the result of her experience working with her clients over the course of 20+ years and living holistically herself in pursuit of ever improving health, wholeness, truth, and authenticity.

With this understanding of how overwhelming some of her suggestions may seem, Fravarti has outlined a 12-week, step-by-step life change program.

While achievement of all her recommendations may take time, any changes that can be made will gradually lead to health improvement and increased vitality. Those who come close to all she proposes experience a swifter healing and recognition of their health goals.

Some of her beliefs that encourage this approach to health care include the idea that every crisis, on any body level, is an opportunity for growth, healing and evolution towards greater health and wholeness. Fravarti often sees people following this path will encounter unanticipated gifts for different body levels. These gifts are often fulfillment of life long dreams. Whether the gift is relief of anxiety, a more balanced emotional state, or the resolution of a persistent problem, these life changes provide the person doing the healing work the encouragement and sustenance they need to continue on their path. She also believes solutions for all areas of life are most often found in the natural changes we can make that will support our body and mind in doing what it is naturally inclined to do....heal itself.

This book outlines a new way of living and looking at health that is not a passive pursuit, which many of us have become accustomed to while operating within the traditional medical system. In western medicine, pills and diagnosis are handed out left and right leaving us to feel personally powerless in the face of any health issue. Live with it, ride it out, 'it's just the way it is' is often the verdict that is recited to the patient. Alternatively, Fravarti offers a path that is empowering and offers the hope of healing and permanent cure. The good news/bad news is that YOU are responsible. This can feel heavy with personal responsibility bearing down OR it can uplift you with the idea that "Yes! There is something I can do!" It's all a matter of perspective and being open to how involved we want to be in the improvement of our health and life.

If you have been seeking personal healing, this book is for you. If you have felt discouraged and lost while you are seeking answers to either simple or deeply concerning health issues, this book is for you. It can work together with whatever other health endeavors you may be pursuing. It will outline support for you on every level of your being, lifting you up to a place of wisdom and confidence while you do your work to heal yourself.

Michele Bryan
Parenting Educator, Author

PREFACE

The motivation for this book came to me as I sought to find answers to the dilemma described by doctor Samuel Hahnemann, the founder of homeopathy. He said he could match the action of the homeopathic remedies so as to provide the stimulus to cure the body of its disease. He went on to say that he was, however, prevented from doing so because the patient could not endure the cure. The movement of the disease in the body (from deeper more critical organs, to less critical and to the surface), in the direction of cure, produces an aggravation of symptoms due to that movement that may include fever, swelling, pain and outbreaks on the skin in the process of healing.

This was the reason for suppressive medicine in the first place. It was meant to provide some measure of relief from suffering when cure appeared not to be a real option. Integrative medicine has advanced two hundred years since Hahnemann's insights about what humans can and can't endure in the name of health and wellness. We now have much to offer the patient to support them through the challenges they may encounter in pursuit of optimal health. Intravenous therapies with vitamin C, calcium disodium EDTA, ALA and ozone have proven profoundly beneficial in support of exactly those patients Hahnemann would have despaired of healing.

Hyperbaric oxygen, osteopathic adjustments and modern chelation therapies often provide an answer to the dilemma of patients otherwise unable to endure the cure. In our time, we can do so much more to support the patient and promote healing than was available to Dr. Hahnemann on behalf of his patients. Laser therapies, orthomolecular therapies and super nutritional therapies together with somatic movement therapies, body mind therapies and biofeedback have all changed the landscape of possibilities we now have that we can bring to bear against the challenge and obstacles to optimal wellness.

The many suggestions in this book are often based on the ideal of restoring new born physiology, as fully as possible, to promote healing. Healthy babies heal very quickly compared to the rest of the population. The efficiency and effectiveness of the healing process in their young bodies is due to the internal environment of optimal pH (6.8) and hydration (72%) together with minimal toxic burden and maximum vital force. We can accelerate the rate at which the body heals itself by speaking the body's language to switch on the kinds of rapid healing that are normally present at birth. This approach explores possibilities of integrating various therapeutic modalities to provide holistic support for deep healing and speedy recovery from many common challenges of our time. This method of co-operation with the natural processes and real needs of the body, at all levels, including psychologically and spiritually, is the intention and orientation behind these guidelines for natural healing.

The ideas that have come together to form this book have emerged from thousands of conversations with clients and from the readings I have done for them as a medical intuitive. This book contains the information I need to accurately guide my clients through the challenges of natural healing and sustainable health. The information contained in these pages is meant to provide educational guidelines for medical professionals, students of natural healing, and for individuals and families who are taking personal responsibility for the kind of health and health care that seems best to them. This book by itself cannot be used to accurately diagnose or treat illness or disease.

The information presented in these pages represents the outlook of an experienced and highly trained intuitive health consultant. It does not represent the outlook that is held by either modern medicine or modern science in some cases and it's not meant to. It's intended to provide alternatives to more conventional but limited ways of thinking. It's meant to provide options in addition to medical treatments that can help create a better outcome for millions of people who have not gotten the health and stamina they need through the many approaches they may have tried so far.

The information and outlook in this book is not new. I have been disseminating this information for many years and have been influenced to do so by those who have gone before me. Doctors, scientists, researchers and leading world experts on sustainability are all contributing their insights, training and specialized skills to solve the problems of our time and create sustainability globally for our mother planet and for the myriad expressions of life that she sustains. Every time I discovered something new about health, wellness and sustainability, I soon learned that others already knew this information. It seems I wasn't first with any of the insights about what works but the contribution of this book is to organize that information and make it available in a clear and convenient form that would provide answers about healing. Available natural therapies are improving faster than our collective health is breaking down. Some of these therapies have proven so effective that they are becoming widely available and thus changing the standards of prevailing practice in all fields of medicine.

THE FIRST STEPS

After consulting for thousands of clients as a homeopath, midwife and guide to natural, safe, effective therapies, I became increasingly aware of the patterns that were emerging from the body of information as a whole. The extensive collection of consultations revealed that certain physiological parameters of hydration, pH, toxic burden, stress and physical fitness would optimize each person's possibilities for safe, effective and permanent healing.

Anyone who succeeds at keeping certain of the body's physiological functions within optimal range will be providing for the body exactly what it needs to accomplish its prime objective: self repair, healing, strength and resilience. Each of the relevant topics of what optimizes and what inhibits the body's healing abilities is explored in a very concise way, short and to the point, so that the reader can learn to do what works with almost absolute certainty.

Each of the subjects introduced in this book could be (and has been) expanded into a full book (or many books) on just that subject. This is a condensed version that will allow readers to benefit from the broad base of expertise while highlighting the keynotes of the most significant and effective considerations. Discover exactly what you need to know about how to get the body's remarkable healing powers to support the accomplishment of your healing and health goals.

Live longer, better and for less, by applying these insights and avoid the common issues of our time that are contributing overwhelming consequences for all of humanity. Diet, hydration, physical fitness and stress reduction all need to be optimized to support the powerhouse of healing that naturally exists in the body. After establishing the guidelines for these most basic healing modalities, the book delves deeper into the healing process through all the major organs and systems of the body. Finally, the consciousness of healing and what supports it is exquisitely explored.

Happiness creates health and supports more rapid healing. Tools and insights for optimizing the healing power of consciousness are written into every page.

HYDRATION

At birth, our bodies are approximately 72% water. That amount steadily decreases over time to about 50% at the time of death from old age or chronic disease. Water molecules are transported through the essential fatty acid cell membrane through protein channels called aqua-porins. The purer the water (less solutes), the higher the osmotic drive to move it into the cells. Hydration very quickly affects the brain, clarity of mental function, and levels of anxiety. Water is the delivery system for oxygen (& other nutrients) to the cells and increases the metabolic rate by supplying the needed base materials for metabolic functions. Increased hydration accelerates metabolism. Water filled foods such as natural fruits and vegetables (unprocessed) are metabolized or digested and assimilated and excreted more easily by the body than are the drying foods which require much more water than they contain in order to metabolize.

One of the most persistent vulnerabilities that I see in the thousands of readings that I do is chronic subclinical dehydration. This is dehydration such that simply drinking water does not resolve it and produce subsequent hydration in short order. In fact, it would be reasonable to call chronic dehydration the crisis of our age and one of the most important problems to solve. There are several causes at work behind this picture of dehydration and in most cases, more than one cause can be found. One of the most widely recognized emergent causes of dehydration is the food supply. Processed foods that are many months old when consumed and that contain rancid oils and are basically non-nutritive, non-life sustaining, dead foods as well as the issues presented by GMO foods which are now present in about 70% of the American food products available in the market place. GMO foods including corn, soy, wheat, rice, canola oil, soybean oil, and cottonseed oil all contain systemic herbicide (glyphosate) in every cell of the final product. BT potatoes are engineered to contain pesticide in every cell and their toxicity is not reduced by peeling or boiling. HFCS is also a product of GMO grain (corn) and has been shown to have debilitating effects on the liver and to block the brain /appetite hormone leptin. Industrial dairy now contains toxic additives of hormones and antibiotics and industrial meats are fed GMO grains full of these herbicides with which the crops were sprayed and they develop diseases that require widespread use of antibiotics. There are also carcinogenic growth hormones used to speed up the animals development for market.

These factors together have helped to create a Standard American Diet that reads -4.2 for us (which means that it harms us continuously) because it metabolizes as 30% sugar and 20% protein and produces an acid pH in the body which uses more hydration than an alkaline pH. For instance, a pH of 5.4 in the body requires about 5 cups more hydration per day than a pH of 6.8. Having a state of metabolic acidosis in the body puts a tremendous extra burden on the kidneys as well. Because it is the kidney's job to keep the blood pH between 7.364 and 7.365, the closer to 7 that we can keep the general body pH, the more we take the burden off the kidneys and help to maintain healthy hydration and support more efficient detoxing of the body. What is needed is a diet that will metabolize as 30% protein and less than 10% sugar because this will dramatically lower cortisol levels, improve hydration and support better cognitive function. Excess cortisol or cortisol flooding due to stress is one of the leading causes of dehydration today because it uses up 4 to 5 cups of additional hydration daily to protect the brain and neurons from cortisol flooding. Being anxious and stressed raises cortisol and burns up hydration. Between elevated cortisol and acidosis, the body may need as much as 9 additional cups of hydration daily added on to the traditional 8 cups of water a day needed to support the body's normal physiological functions. It's not really possible to drink 16 or more cups of water per day and a situation of water debt develops in the body. The fatty acid membrane covering each cell becomes sclerosed, hardened, and toughened and the osmotic processes are impeded and become more sluggish, less efficient. Nutrient assimilation and distribution is impaired and the cells become congested, unable to detox, to transport oxygen and maintain vitality. It can take many weeks to reverse a water debt, even months, and it takes more than just drinking water to reverse chronic dehydration.

A rehydration protocol usually includes raw juice (3 cups daily), high protein broth (2 to 3 cups daily), fresh ginger tea (3 cups daily) because it helps raise pH and structured water because it hydrates twice as efficiently as any other water. Rehydration also requires of us the discipline of an elimination diet. Avoiding drying and dehydrating foods is a wiser choice than trying to compensate for the detrimental effects of these ersatz foods. For the most part, the focus of what to eliminate can be summed up as grains, rancid oils, chocolate and processed convenience foods. It is possible to create with these guidelines a personal diet that reads +4 or better and that is always healing you rather than submitting to the American diet of depleted, chemicalized processed foods that is hurting us with every bite.

Dehydrating Foods

Juice, especially reconstituted
Coffee, tea, sodas
Alcohol
Artificial sweeteners, high fructose corn syrup
Sugar, honey, salt
Hydrogenated oils, also rancid oils

Candy, ice cream
Deli meats, salami, processed lunch meats, hot dogs, sausage, ham
Fish containing mercury, lead, arsenic or cadmium
Dry roasted salted nuts
Fried pork rinds, cheese puffs
Chips, especially if made with GMO grains, contain rancid oils or lots of additives/ flavorings
Popcorn, especially with movie butter topping

Dry Foods

Bread, bagels, biscuits, muffins, croissants, crackers, burger and hot dog buns
Pancakes, waffles, pasta, pizza
Pastry, cakes, cookies, donuts
French fries, onion rings
Meal replacement bars, protein bars, granola bars
Processed cheese including American, Velveeta, Cheez Whiz, Nacho Cheese toppings,
Meat from animals fed GMO foods and pesticide laced grains and treated with hormones and antibiotics

Instead of these food substitutes that we have become culturally accustomed to that profoundly deplete us and do nothing to support our health and vitality, we need to be eating a more non-processed and more substantially raw food diet. A diet composed of 70% raw foods and about 30% protein is ideal for healing the human body in most cases. The young people of today are especially embracing the raw food movement and are largely responsible for it's ever increasing popularity. Eating a diet of very healthy food on a daily basis can take up to one third of our time, energy and resources to shop, plan and prepare, and it is for this reason that the insidious convenience foods have literally taken over. By sacrificing your health to the convenience food diet you can put your energy, time and resources into other goals, but at what cost, ultimately?

Rehydrating Foods

Whole natural fruits and vegetables, especially raw juice
Watermelon, grapes
Raw nuts and seeds, especially when soaked (nut cream)
Natural dry fruits including dates, raisins, apricots, cherries and pineapple
Whole organic milks and cheeses
Organic eggs
Cooked grains - oats, rice, beans, cream of wheat, grits, couscous
Natural fresh meats, poultry and fish (of which there is very little in your market place)

Soups and broths
Agave nectar - in small amounts as a low glycemic sweetener for ginger tea
Fresh ginger tea, agua frescas, herbal teas
Homemade slow food from whole organic unprocessed ingredients

In 1828, Americans consumed an average of 12 pounds of sugar per year. In the 1890's the introduction of Cola's into the culture (which became immediately popular) and the abundance of refined white flour and processed foods became the foundation of the junk food industry which is to this day incredibly profitable. By 1928, statistics indicate that Americans were consuming twice as much sugar as 100 years before, averaging 24 pounds per person annually. By 1975, per person consumption of sugar and corn syrup sweeteners had risen to 124 pounds per year. By 1999, the statistic had risen to 158 pounds per person. That translates to roughly one third of consumed calories coming directly from sweeteners and another third of calories coming from refined carbohydrates which also metabolize as glucose.

Together this produces a very high level of insulin - the sugar metabolizing, fat producing hormone, and eventually it produces Insulin Resistance and Type 2 Diabetes. These are not real foods. They are fake foods, ersatz foods, and they comprise two thirds of our diet, sometimes more. These foods fill us and bloat us but leave us hungry even as the excess glucose is being converted to glycogen and stored as fat. Fat, but metabolically starving due to empty calories, we cannot eat enough to fill the emptiness inside. We become addicted to food and to over eating.

Choosing to drink only water is one of the best and simplest choices one can make to protect your health. Blessing the water you drink helps even more. If you choose to consume dehydrating foods and non-foods, you can help protect yourself to some degree by offsetting the negative effects by compensating with the best super saturating water (Penta) daily in liberal quantities.

Rehydration is also a spiritual challenge in that a critical outlook uses hydration, and learning to overcome judgmental tendencies keeps us better hydrated. Being unhappy uses more hydration than being happy. Being anxious and worried uses more hydration than being calm and relaxed. Staying habitually stressed as a lifestyle and outlook choice may support certain types of worldly accomplishments, pushing us in the direction of our goals, but that will always need to be tempered with some form of Sabbath (a form of calm repose that manifests being without efforting), if the body is to enjoy it's full potential of vitality and resilience. Resilience is a quality of water. My teacher, the sufi mystic Hazrat Inayat Khan, said that water performs the same function in this plane that love performs in the higher planes. I find that it is the water in the cells of the body that allow one to hold the resonance of their spiritual practice and be less reactive to circumstantial challenges. Water in the body, in every cell of the body, is holding the resonance of innocence, of purity, of childlike enthusiasm and of optimism.

The leading sign of dehydration, (the first to appear), is anxiety, concern, worry, fear, stress. In America, when we find ourselves overwhelmed by these challenges we are offered a prescription medication to help us cope. This medication also is a source of dehydration if used daily long term. Thus our medicine becomes our poison and our problem becomes worse by the very means we use to relieve it. Instead of an anxiety medication, most of us would do much better and get more relief if we choose just to have the glass of water and re-find our balance by observing our life carefully and doing what works, balancing activity with repose, and choosing more of what fills us with life, optimism and enthusiasm and less of what robs us and depletes us of those life affirming energies.

Causes Of Dehydration

Diet, highly refined, processed foods, convenience foods, rancid oils
Chemicals and food additives and pesticide residues
Medications, prescription and nonprescription including steroids, pain relievers, anti-depressants, statins, anti-hypertensives, antibiotics, cold and flu medicines
Inadequate Fluid intake, limited consumption of water - at especially high risk are the mentally disabled, autistics, brain injury, mentally ill or depressed, teenagers and the elderly, none of whom are fully capable of understanding their water needs.
Illness, Chronic and Acute including vomiting, fever, diarrhea, inflammation, Meningitis and Encephalitis, Diabetes
Renal/Adrenal Insufficiency, nephrosis, kidney diseases, adrenal exhaustion
Sodium retention/edema, congestive heart disease
Liver Diseases, Cirrhosis, hepatitis
Trauma, physical and psychological
Stress especially chronic high stress

Severe dehydration, including subclinical chronic dehydration is usually accompanied by acidosis. Metabolic acidosis eventually impairs brain functions by disrupting the acetyl choline cycle of the brain and reduces mental clarity, ultimately producing dementia or senility. To metabolize what we consume and adequately rehydrate the body often takes far more water than we think. The following list gives some guidelines for using water to offset other choices and produce a sustainable outcome.

To metabolize & rehydrate: Takes this much water or Penta

8 oz. coffee with 1 1/2 tsp. sugar	30 oz	15 oz.
1 Starbucks Carmel Macchiato, Venti	38 oz.	18 oz.
6 oz. wine	30 oz.	15 oz.
1 margarita	60 oz.	30 oz.
12 oz. beer	38 oz.	18 oz.
16 oz. soda with corn syrup sweetener	57 oz.	27 oz.
16 oz. soda, artificial sweetener	63 oz.	32 oz.
8 oz. corn syrup sweetened candy	35 oz.	18 oz.
8 oz. chocolate/corn syrup candy	42 oz.	20 oz.
2 oz. pancake/waffle syrup (artificial flavor)	22 oz.	12 oz.
2 oz. pure maple syrup	20 oz.	10 oz.
2 oz. agave sweetener	8 oz.	4 oz.
8 oz. sweetened cereal	35 oz.	17 oz.
8 oz. rbGH milk	20 oz.	9 oz.
8 ounces whole organic milk	12 oz	7 oz.
8 oz. orange juice from concentrate	48 oz	20 oz.
8 oz. fresh squeezed orange juice	13 oz	6 oz.
2 oz. processed nacho cheese topping	30 oz.	13 oz.
1 oz. canola oil	26 oz.	12 oz.
1 oz. virgin olive oil	4 oz.	2 oz.
1 dose of Ambien or Zyrtec	40 oz.	20 oz.
1 dose Valium, Zanax, Paxil, Celexa	28 oz.	12 oz.
1 dose OxyContin, Percocet	38 oz.	20 oz.
1 dose NyQuil or DayQuil	48 oz.	25 oz.
1 large tub movie popcorn with butter topping	38 oz.	18 oz.
Add a large drink for an additional	100 oz.	40 oz.
Those last two together	18 cups	7 cups

pH - Potential Of Hydrogen, In Solution

On the pH scale the more hydrogen ions, the more acidic, the less hydrogen ions the more alkaline. The critical blood pH of the human body is 7.35 to 7.45, slightly alkaline. To maintain this alkalinity of the blood, the body adjusts the urine pH through the kidney function increasing urine acidity to preserve blood alkalinity. Acid pH means increased excretion of hydrogen ions by the kidneys. It also means increased excretion of potassium ions and increased ammonia in the urine. The excess acid also goes into the interstitial fluids, the fluid between the cells. Lymphatic functions which take place in the fluid between the cells are thereby disrupted. The pancreas, liver and gall bladder are overtaxed in the production of alkalizing enzymes and digestive and assimilation functions weaken. A chronic state of acidosis causes calcium to be leached from the bones to act as a buffering agent. Acidosis stimulates overproduction of insulin, the fat storage hormone, promoting weight gain.

Inadequate fluid intake further inhibits the body's alkalizing processes by preventing optimum kidney function and detoxing of the body's tissues.

An average urine pH below 6 is too acidic. Ideal is 6.5 to 7. A urine pH of 5.2 is a state of acidosis which will produce biochemical anomalies throughout the body, including disturbances in the acetylcholine cycle in the brain. This deficiency of neuro-nutrients is a factor in cognitive decline and dementia. Chronic subclinical dehydration also disrupts the GABA cycle in the brain producing panic attacks and chronic anxiety.

Prescriptions for mood altering drugs further dehydrate the body (or require increased fluid intake) and they contribute to the toxic burden in solution which further acidifies the body. Well known alkalizers include lots of pure fresh water, whole fresh raw foods and lemon juice in water.

Whether the body is acid or alkaline determines whether it is in a catabolic state which produces degeneration of cells, tissues, organs and systems or whether the body is in an anabolic state which produces regeneration. The pH of the body is negatively affected by stress and toxic thoughts which raise cortisol levels and use up hydration. PH is also affected by activity level, exercise and metabolic functions and the acid condition of the body causes retention of fat to buffer the chemical imbalance. Energy production at the level of cell respiration is the source of the acid alkaline balance. Cells excrete metabolic waste that is acidic. Any food that has a high glycemic index, which includes all processed grains, is considered acid forming. Artificial sweeteners are even more acid forming than sugar.

It is the pH balance in the body's fluids and tissues which allow for the production of oxygen and the assimilation of nutrients. Absorption of vitamins and minerals, particularly calcium, is blocked by excess acid pH.

pH - Degenerative Disease

The degenerative diseases produced or promoted by acid pH and relieved by alkaline pH include: thyroid diseases, bone disease, including arthritis and osteoporosis, muscle wasting, soreness & cramps including fibromyalgia, circulatory problems, diabetes, and cancer. Acid pH inhibits the production of dopamine which has a major role in pain control. For a patient with fibromyalgia, more acidic means less dopamine and more pain. Stress and overactivity contribute to the acid imbalance just about equally to consumption of an acid forming diet.

Respiratory disease is also a significant contributor to acidosis. As much as one third of the acid alkaline balance is regulated by respiration. When gaseous exchange is impaired and a state of hypoxia (low oxygen) exists, as happens with advancing emphysema, a state of respiratory acidosis develops. When diffusion of respiratory gases is reduced due to asthma or sleep apnea, respiratory acidosis also develops.

Different tissues of the body have vastly different pH to support their various functions. The stomach, for instance has a very low acid pH (5.3) because that is what is necessary for the breakdown of foods. The thyroid, by comparison, has a very high pH (8.3) because the parathyroid glands embedded in the thyroid tissue are responsible for the uptake and release of calcium and the determination of whether to lay down this element for the mineralization of bones and teeth or to pull calcium from storage in bone and muscle cells and return it to the circulation to buffer acidosis. The three critical factors which most determine health are pH, hydration and stress. Acid pH has long been identified as a risk factor for the development of abnormal cells in the body. Better pH balance improves oxygenation, metabolism, nutrition and cognitive function. Smoking, alcohol, and chemicals are acid forming.

Fresh pure water, raw foods, exercise including yoga and walking as well as meditation and prayer all are alkalizing to the body.

FOOD POWER

Food is the power source for the human body. The Standard American diet today (2018) reads -4.2 for us. That diet hurts us with every bite. It is quite possible to create a diet that reads +4 for us, but it is a change of outlook that is required to do so. The modern American diet metabolizes at an average of 30% sugar and 20% protein. Even protein powders, a highly refined processed food supplement, metabolize at about 28% sugar and 20% protein. A therapeutic diet to support healing needs to be closer to 10% sugar and 30% protein. The average diet in America is currently 3 to 4% raw food and 93% processed foods. This diet dehydrates the body and changes the pH from alkaline to acid. Optimal pH in the human body is 6.8 to 7 but the average pH of our bodies is now 5.4, a significant state of acidosis. The fastest way to change an acid pH to alkaline is raw unprocessed food. Changing the diet to about 70% raw will, in most cases, change the pH to about 6.8 which is ideal for prevention of cancer, heart disease, fibromyalgia, arthritis and dementia. There is a profound effect upon the kidneys when the pH is maintained as close as possible to 7 because it takes a burden off and allows for efficient detoxing. The kidneys are responsible for keeping the blood pH at 7.364 and we can either strengthen them or weaken them in this ability by what we consume. The extra burden on the kidneys of acid pH eventually results in renal hypertension.

The human body is a protein based machine and every action in every cell of the body is regulated by the actions of proteins. A therapeutic diet intended to rebuild strength and resilience or support recovery of stamina and vitality needs to metabolize as 30% protein. This high level of protein will significantly lower cortisol levels and thus support hydration. Rather than recommend consumption of additional whole meats which may burden the digestive system and make it sluggish and inefficient, it is wiser to supplement with several cups of high protein broth daily. In this form the protein will be more easily assimilated and available to the body with less demand on the digestive powers than is the case with whole meat. However, I am referring to homemade broth that you make up in your crock pot at home, fresh every few days and not to a processed broth that you buy at the market as a convenience. The difference between these two forms of broth in terms of how they support the body is almost beyond belief. The best processed broth in the marketplace is going to read zero (meaning it does no harm) and the homemade broth is going to read +8 or even +9 on a ten point scale of relative benefit for the body when particularly well matched to the individual needs. This high protein broth can be bone marrow, beef broth, lamb, chicken or turkey, or fish broth. Use high quality fresh whole ingredients and let simmer in the crock pot over night or for about 10 to 12 hours.

For a strict vegan diet, the best protein super food is soaked nuts, especially almond cream made from raw almonds soaked for 30 hours. Soaking increases the protein content by as much as 300% and makes it more digestible and also increases the availability of the Omega 3's and 6's making it a perfect brain food. A vegan diet will assimilate at about 24% protein if nut cream is consumed on a near daily basis, such as added to raw juices and as dressing on salads. My teacher, the Sufi Master and Mystic Hazrat Inayat Khan, told a story that I discovered somewhere in the course of my training, that has been profoundly supportive to me. He said that spiritual legend tells that Lord Sri Shiva required of his disciples that they should eat meat if they in any way heard or saw or seemed to perceive what others did not. If they had any super sensory perception, they also had, according to Lord Shiva, the weakest of constitutions and would therefore not be able to withstand the rigors of training as his disciple, if they refused to eat meat (as was the Brahmin tradition of many of these young men). This helped me to choose a diet that made me strong and capable and hearty rather than one which made me spiritually pure but fragile. For me this turned out to be no real problem as in my case, staying spiritually pure is much simpler and easier to accomplish than staying physically strong.

Buying processed foods from a natural market does not ensure a good diet. Processed foods, even protein powders, metabolize as higher sugar (28-30%) and lower protein (18-20%). Yes, even the very best protein powders, even the raw ones, because they are processed, highly refined and at least several months old and they metabolize differently than whole fresh foods. Learning to prepare raw foods that are fresh and natural and appealing seems to some like an affront to the American entitlement of convenience, but convenience foods are most destructive to our well being. They are really food substitutes, substances that will look and taste like foods but that will not feed us.

Modern industrial dairy is one of the processed convenience foods that we have become dependent upon. This is not the same dairy, ounce for ounce, as the dairy products that were the standard of 50 years ago. It has been depleted of much of its nutritive value while its toxic burden seems to be increasing exponentially. Food that was until recently highly nutritious and safe has been changed through modern industrial agriculture and food processing standards to a product that in many cases is not even safe, much less beneficial. Non-dairy processed cheeses, like soy cheese, are not nutritionally sound either. This highly refined processed soy has been subjected to such extremes of heat and pressure in order to produce the desired cheese-like texture and consistency that the human body will be entirely unable to break the molecular bond thus created and the ersatz cheese food product will benefit the body to about the same degree as eating the plastic wrapper.

Soy milk and almond milk have become popular substitutes for those wishing to avoid the problems that are associated with dairy. They generally taste appealing and serve the purpose of convenience but they are not real foods. Homemade, fresh almond milk made from raw soaked almonds (x 30 hrs) will generally read at +9.3 beneficial, essentially a superfood. Babies can thrive on it. The industrially produced almond milk available in your market place may be up to six months old and will generally read about -3.2 or slightly harmful to the human body.

Processed food is an addiction to convenience that comes at a high cost. The foods we are depending upon to make our day easier are actually making our days much harder by robbing us of strength, resilience, vitality and even cognitive function. Yes, that means that eating a diet comprised largely of highly refined processed convenience foods effectively lowers functional intelligence by disrupting the acetyl choline cycle of the brain through acidosis and chronic subclinical dehydration. Eating whole unprocessed and raw foods will make one both stronger and smarter than eating a diet of refined cereals and processed dairy.

What to eat and what to drink quickly becomes an urgent question when trying to reduce the amount of processed food in the diet. It can be very helpful to design a basic support system that provides super nutrition, alkaline pH and adequate hydration so that the processed food one does get is within the body's range for coping with the challenge. Fresh homemade ginger tea with a pH of 9 is a good staple to add when trying to change the body to a healthier more alkaline pH. Most things one drinks in our culture, including coffee, teas, sodas, alcohol, processed fruit juice, sports drinks, and energy drinks will have an effective metabolic pH of about 3 and will effectively lower the body's pH toward a more acid base. Fresh ginger root purchased from the market, peeled, chopped and simmered, strained and diluted, makes a refreshing beverage that counters the pervasive tendency to acidosis inherent in the modern American diet. Also, water with lemon can serve a similar function, helping to detox the kidneys and better support rehydration through more ideal pH balance. In fact, all citrus helps support alkaline pH. The most alkalizing foods are ginger, lemons and limes and avocados. All greens are also beneficial for supporting alkaline pH and cilantro, basil, mint, watercress and spinach are particularly beneficial.

One of the problems associated with the processed convenience foods in our markets is the pervasive presence of high fructose corn syrup. HFCS entered our market on the back of government subsidies in the 1970's and, in part due to this financial advantage, is now present in 70 to 75% of all our processed foods, including many foods we don't think of as sweet such as crackers and breads. HFCS has many properties that make it desirable to the processed food industry such as browning properties, texture and preservative, but most of all, it's just cheap. There is another point of importance about HFCS and that is the way it is metabolized in the body. From the viewpoint of marketing, HFCS is a perfect food because it is almost irresistible and it makes you hungry. HFCS is metabolized in the liver and only the liver. Not one molecule of it reaches the brain as food or energy. Therefore, the brain does not release the hormone leptin indicating that it has been fed. It has not been fed and continues to release hormones to increase appetite. Meanwhile, the body may be stuffed over-full and unable to consume more and yet be starving, at the molecular level, in the physiology of the cells and nutrients to the brain. People eat because they feel hungry. Eating foods that turn off the hunger results in less consumed. Almond cream made from soaked raw almonds supports the brain in several ways including the production of leptin as well as providing the very best source essential fatty acids called omegas. It is a superfood for the brain and it reduces hunger. HFCS actually increases hunger by blocking assimilation of nutrients.

High Fructose Corn Syrup (HFCS) and why is it dangerous?

This product in our food chain begins with Round-up Ready corn or corn which has an herbicide present systemically throughout every cell. This is GMO corn which has been genetically altered so that it can be sprayed with a specific herbicide. The herbicidal chemical is then in every cell of the plant and in the corn. Upon harvesting, this corn is not immediately edible. You cannot pick it, cook it and eat it. Until it is processed, it cannot be eaten by humans. It is, however, fed to our livestock nationwide and is thus causing additional harm elsewhere in the food chain. To make HFCS, the corn is broken down into a mash and mixed with an acid to cause it to further breakdown into high fructose.

In the human body, sugar generally metabolizes as 50% glucose and 50% fructose. The half that metabolizes as glucose feeds the brain and provides energy for the body. Fully half of the product called sugar is usable by the body and usable very quickly, so there is some benefit for the body. Though certainly one can eat too much sugar, this has become much more of a problem since the sweetener has been changed to HFCS.

Now that which is sweet provides no energy and causes an increase of appetite because the brain cannot use it as food. It will be metabolized by the liver as a toxin, the same as alcohol. Repeated and frequent consumption of HFCS will produce a sluggish, congested, fatty liver the same way alcohol will and it frequently results in malnutrition in overweight bodies and diminishing vitality. The same diet which is being fed to feedlot cattle to fatten them quickly for market, a diet which will kill these animals in very short order if they weren't already scheduled for slaughter, is the diet which is being fed to price and convenience conscious middle America and it is doing the same thing to their bodies as it is doing to the cattle.

So, the source of the hidden danger behind HFCS is a GMO crop designed to benefit production and marketing, but that is detrimental to human bodies because it produces acidosis which damages every cell of the body. This product is financially irresistible to the food industry thanks to government subsidies. It is appealing to the consumer in taste and appearance and it has completely changed the American body type in just 35 years. All of the primary GMO crops (corn, soy, wheat, canola) have together been largely responsible for changing the shape of American bodies and a primary reason why we struggle so to keep fit. American wheat and soy are also sprayed with herbicide the same as corn. The wheat and soy is genetically altered to survive the toxic herbicide and then when the crop is sprayed with the chemical cocktail of Round-up, it is contained in every cell of the plant and every grain of wheat and every soybean.

More and more people are discovering that they need to avoid the processed grain products, most of which also contain GMO oils (soy, canola and cottonseed) or else they feel poorly, bloated, uncomfortable, and dim witted. People who were never celiac, who never had any known wheat sensitivity, are now becoming increasingly reactive to the processed grains available in their marketplace and in their restaurants. Loss of I.Q. and cognitive abilities are made worse by a diet of these highly processed fake convenient food substitutes and can be reversed by eliminating these foods. Allergies, sinus infections and food sensitivities are all made worse by processed foods, especially GMO grains and all of those symptoms can be relieved by taking those foods out of the diet.

Therapeutic Diet Guidelines

Daily raw fruit and vegetable juice - 2 to 3 cups, (carrot, apple, spinach for instance, or pineapple, carrot, orange - feel free to add 2 or 3 other juices to any combination according to availability). This helps rehydrate the body and raises the pH to 6.8

Nut cream - 3 to 4 oz. (or 7 to 8 oz. nut milk) daily. This is especially important for vegans and for extra cognitive support and to support the production of leptin. This superfood provides high quality protein and essential fatty acids and makes the raw juice taste fantastic, a true high protein smoothie made entirely raw and unprocessed.

Daily high protein broth - 2 to 3 cups of homemade beef, chicken, turkey or fish broth. This is a superfood of easily assimilated protein and helps support ideal hydration. Keeping the protein proportion of the diet at about 30% builds physical strength and resilience and lowers cortisol levels and thus helps with hydration (because high cortisol uses up lots of hydration). Vegans who do not wish to eat meat broths can increase their protein levels with nut cream and substitute 2 to 3 cups of homemade fresh vegetable broth for support of hydration and for pH balance.

Fresh ginger tea - 2 to 4 cups daily to alkalize the pH and heal the intestinal mucosa. Has an ideal pH for rebalancing from our over acidic diets. Helps promote ideal hydration. Also, lemon water, throughout the day helps detox the kidneys and supports better hydration and pH.

Raw nuts and seeds and dry fruit - for snacks homemade raw trail mix (no chocolate) or bliss balls.

Homemade raw pies and desserts.
Make fresh salad dressings, either lemon and oil or vinegar and oil or nut sauces and dressings.

Dairy - use organic and highest quality in all dairy products. Consider artisanal dairy from local farms or Farmer's markets, goats milk cheeses. Use real butter.

Oils - use highest quality cold pressed oils - olive, sunflower, safflower, almond, walnut, and grape seed oil

Find raw food chefs and look for raw food groups meeting in your community.
Shop Farmer's markets for freshly prepared non-industrial condiments, pickles, jams, wheat free baked goods or higher quality wheat baked goods, grass fed meats and local dairy as well as the best fresh fruits and vegetables.
Avoid HFCS (high fructose corn syrup)
Avoid GMO grains (all sprayed with herbicide)
Avoid soybean oil, canola and cottonseed oil (all GMO and sprayed with herbicide)
Avoid processed foods such as breads, crackers, cereals, chips, pretzels, pasta, pastries, desserts and candy, especially chocolate
Avoid sodas, coffee, alcohol, processed juice, energy drinks and sports drinks (drink water, lemon water or ginger tea)
Avoid fried foods and rancid and heated oils in general
Avoid Dairy containing antibiotics and growth hormones

Healthy Sweet

Our brains have a reward circuitry based on release of dopamine that influences appetite by rewarding increased calorie intake independent of taste as well as rewarding taste, which will signal the brain that increased glucose is available. This brain circuitry encourages the consumption of calories that will quickly raise blood sugar levels. If we did not subsist primarily on processed food, that brain message would serve us very well by guiding us to eat high energy foods like fruits and honey. The sweet foods we would consume in the absence of processed foods would all contain significant trace minerals including magnesium, calcium, iron, and phosphorus as well as anti-oxidant compounds and other nutrients. Those naturally sweet foods provide quick relief for adrenal exhaustion which disrupts the ability to maintain blood glucose levels and they contain food fiber which slows the rate of absorption of the sugars into the blood stream.

Humans have been producing refined sugar for at least 2,000 years. Alexander the Great encountered the marvel of sugar when he arrived in India. Beet sugar, which now comprises about half the processed sugar produced in America, has been manufactured for over 200 years. Sugar did not become a significant health issue until the industrial age invented highly refined processed convenience foods that will feed a work force cheaply and without taking up productive work time. Our addiction to instant cheap food is entirely man-made and it was done primarily for the sake of financial profits. We are being fed cheap sugars to keep us going longer, working unnatural schedules and producing a gross national income that mostly goes into someone else's pockets, not ours.

The artificial food supply is not a response to consumer demand. It is driven by government decisions about what's best for the country relative to world markets and world politics. Crop subsidies that promote the dominance of toxic chemical laden grains in our food supply and then distribute them to the most vulnerable through the national lunch programs continue to destroy the health of the citizens because the government has determined that there are interests at stake which supersede your rights as an individual to health and well being.

In fact, that premise, also exists in the mandate of the national vaccination policies which explicitly state that the individual's right to avoid vaccines that may injure them are superseded by the government's right to protect your neighbors at the expense of your own well being. The individual is expendable, a throwaway commodity in this system of government. This same policy has been reiterated in America's new health care insurance. Under the guise of health care for all, the law specifically states that the decisions are to be based on parameters set by the state and not by the doctor and the needs of the patient he serves.

This change in values relative to health care options emerges directly out of the governments manipulation of the food supply and the subsequent national health crisis produced by the mass consumption of a chemically toxic and non-nutritive diet. America's two year olds are eating 14 teaspoons of sugar each day. Our two year olds are not choosing that diet for themselves. The standard American diet metabolizes at about 30% sugar. This is partly due to the added sugars and HFCS, but it is also due to the fact that all highly refined processed carbohydrates (grains) metabolize as sugar. This diet contains three times the recommended amount of sugar. Recommended by whom? You might well ask. Even the U.S. Department of Agriculture guidelines recommend about two thirds less sugar than the current average. The same government that is subsidizing this unhealthy diet is also telling us we shouldn't eat that diet because it's creating a national epidemic of obesity, diabetes, cancer and heart disease. Sugar itself is not the problem. An abundant supply of cheap, unhealthy food is the problem. Sugars are building blocks in the formation of RNA and DNA. Sugars are even found in interstellar gas clouds and very likely have a role as chemical precursors to the development of life on earth.

When Did Sweet Become Unhealthy?

Consumption of HFCS has come to dominate the current market of industrial age sweeteners. HFCS is not metabolized in the body the same as sugar despite advertising claims to the contrary.

For instance, HFCS fails to trigger the production of the brain hormone leptin. The function of leptin is to acknowledge being fed and supply an appetite suppressant to signal satiation and absence of hunger. The result is one can gorge themselves, massively overeating to the point of physical discomfort and yet still feel hungry. Really hungry. Thus the body's appetite is manipulated to far exceed its capacity to process what is consumed.

Secondly, HFCS is a carrier for the toxin glyphosate because it is made from GMO corn that is sprayed with this herbicide. The way that our immune systems are compromised by the high sugar diet renders our bodies less capable of eliminating this toxin which is processed by the liver and eliminated through the colon. Though HFCS is the most widely used artificial sweetener, there are now many more. Unlike HFCS, which came into wide spread use because government subsidies made it cheap, other artificial sweeteners have gained a place in the market because they add no substantial calories and they are exponentially sweeter than sugar. These chemical sweeteners are being challenged on the basis of their ability to disrupt normal metabolic processes because they are 200, 700 and even up to 20,000 times sweeter than natural foods.

The Current Artificial Sweeteners In Widespread Use Are:

Saccharin - called Sweet and Low reads -4.2 for kidney damage
Aspartame - called Equal and NutraSweet -3.6 for nervous system and brain, and reads -4.2 for kidneys
Sucralose - called Splenda (was accidentally discovered in the process of creating an insecticide) reads -4.2 for kidneys
Neotame - called Newtame, reads -3.4 for kidneys
Acesulfame - potassium, called Sweet One, reads -4.2 for nervous system
A new artificial sweetener has just received FDA approval as a food additive that may be used to sweeten soft drinks, jams and jellies, syrups and baked goods. The newest addition is called **Advantame** and is the sweetest chemical yet at about 20,000 times sweeter than sugar. It reads -4.2 for the digestive system, small and large intestines.

The motivation behind choosing no calorie sweeteners is the idea of all the pleasure with none of the weight gain. The reality has turned out to be that artificial sweeteners are making people fat. One reason seems to be the increase in consumption overall, relative to consumption of sugar sweetened calories. The sugar turns off the appetite, whereas artificial sweeteners do not. The reward circuitry of the brain is triggered by caloric intake independent of taste so the brain prefers sugar over non-caloric sweeteners and the brain releases dopamine in response to sugar but not in response to the "diet" sweeteners. Sugar sends the signal to stop eating. High fructose and artificial sweeteners do not.

Natural Sweeteners

honey - ranges from zero for processed to +4.2 for Manuka honey
dates, fruit - ranges from +5 to +7
agave - reads zero, neutral
molasses - zero
rice syrup - zero
barley malt - zero
maple syrup range - zero to +4
organic white sugar - zero
organic brown sugar - zero
stevia - zero, safest sweetener for diabetics
xylitol - zero, positive as tooth protectant, not for baking

When it comes to sweet, raw natural and unprocessed is best for health.

Raw honey - is a positive choice as are dates and other fruits. Date sugar is more processed than dates. Maple syrup is a good natural sweetener and it metabolizes better than agave. Agave, however, is still one of the safe sweeteners. It is a highly refined processed sugar, but it has a higher glycemic index than sugar which means it metabolizes more slowly and doesn't raise blood sugar levels as quickly. Agave is also sweeter than sugar and attains the same effective sweetness with 30% less. Which is to say that sugar would require 30% more in amount to equal the sweetness attained with agave. A clear advantage.

Brown rice syrup and barley malt syrup - are also lower glycemic natural sweeteners however, they are not nearly as sweet and require considerably larger quantities to satisfactorily sweeten recipes.

Stevia - a non caloric but highly processed sweetener (turning green leaves into white powder is processing) that is a safe choice for those with insulin resistance or diabetes.

Homemade treats often read zero for us, or neutral and safe which is preferable to the negative 8 and 9 of many processed confections. Making your own homemade from the best ingredients or buying from artisanal cooks producing the highest quality fresh product is always better than cheap treats of candy, cookies, sodas and other non-nutritive fake foods. Homemade treats can be loaded with nutritional value that is missing from convenience foods with a long shelf life. Homemade bliss balls made from raw nuts and dried fruits read plus 9, which makes dessert more supportive to health than most of the meal.

We can make healthy sustainable choices and still have desserts and treats everyday if we make them from healthy ingredients. We cannot make a boxed cake mix with canned frosting other than about negative 9 as to how it's processed in the body. Take the convenience foods out. Grind your own raw nuts and rolled oats to make gluten free flour. Use organic free range eggs and whole butter. Use healthy butter or organic cream cheese to make the frosting and you've eliminated all the chemicals, the preservatives, the colorings, and the rancid oils and produced real food that will read about +4 or even higher instead of the non-nutritive fake foods that have taken over our diet.

If your sweet cravings are overwhelming, you may get significant relief by increasing your protein. Eating healthy protein at every meal helps stabilize blood sugar levels in a healthy range and provides longer lasting energy stores to support the days activities. Reducing overall carbohydrates like breads, pasta and cereals together with increased protein will improve adrenal support. The adrenals have a very important role in balancing blood sugar. Adrenal support in the form of stress relief together with adequate protein and vitamin C will improve vitality and resilience and reduce sugar cravings.

Dairy And Non-Dairy Substitutes

Unhealthy dairy and unhealthy dairy substitutes should be eliminated and replaced with healthier options that still provide the comfort and culinary creativity to enhance our enjoyment and create health. I use the term 'Industrial dairy' to indicate unhealthy dairy and I compare that to organic dairy, artisanal dairy and fresh nut milks. Artisanal dairy refers to raw milk dairy and goat milk, both of which produce much healthier cheeses than the cheaper industrial dairy cheese.

America's dairy products are designed for long shelf life. Expiration dates on milk are up to 5 weeks after production. Fresh food consumed within days of being produced is best for health, but the longest possible shelf life is always best for profits. Many delightfully fresh and nutritious dairy foods are available at farmer's markets.

Next after the local farmer's market, highest quality imported cheese from France, Ireland or Switzerland is a better quality of food than cheaper processed cheeses. Usually, even the healthiest dairy options only read zero or neutral at best, meaning, safe to include in the diet but not beneficial. However, in most cases, a therapeutic diet does not include any dairy other than butter and ghee.

Non-dairy milk - is only an improvement over unhealthy dairy products when the non-dairy substitute is fresh homemade from the finest ingredients such as raw almonds and structured water and medjool dates for sweetening. The dairy substitutes that are packaged in aseptic containers and sitting on the market shelf for 8 months always read negative for everyone. Processed rice milk, soy milk and almond milk read negative five to negative nine on a scale of food choices, whereas fresh homemade almond milk reads positive nine and homemade rice milk reads neutral / safe. Homemade fresh soy milk still reads slightly negative and is not recommended, but the processed versions in the market place are 300% worse.

Rice milk - is usually made from brown rice. Research has recently shown that arsenic levels are much higher in brown rice and many brown rice products including baby food were found to have shockingly high concentrations of arsenic. Rice milk is usually chosen because of known sensitivities to dairy and soy. These highly allergic types usually thrive on fresh almond milk, but processed rice milk should not be considered a safer choice. Rice milk is low protein and high carbohydrate.

Soy milk - is represented as having an excellent nutritional profile with high protein, low saturated fat and no cholesterol, but soy has not lived up to the promises that are made in its name. Soy has proved to be an endocrine disrupter in the human body mimicking the effects of certain hormones and contributing to further hormone imbalance. Soy protein is difficult to digest. In its natural state it is suitable only for ruminants, animals with more than one stomach. In its highly refined processed state it metabolizes as 26 to 29% sugar and no more than 20% protein and it is guaranteed to lower your pH and hydration, further weakening digestion functions. This is not real food. Because most people don't enjoy the flavor of soy, sweeteners and flavors including chocolate are added to make it more palatable. Without the marketing, no one would drink soy milk based on its own merits. Soy cheese is about as digestible as the plastic wrapper it comes in. Raw goat cheese is usually a better option or a homemade nut cheese for vegans.

Almond milk - almonds are a super food providing high protein and beneficial essential fatty acids, but processed almond milk does not deliver the benefits of raw soaked almonds. Processed almond milk is low in protein because it is mostly sweetened water. It tastes good, it's low in calories and it's vegan, but the processed version that is already many months old when you pick it up from the grocery shelf is not a real food, whereas, the natural fresh homemade form is one of the best foods available for brain health, heart health and vitality. Fine mesh bags for straining fresh nut milk are available at purejoyplanet.com

Processed hemp milk - is not a good option and neither are processed coconut milk and processed coconut water. None of these products deliver the health and nutrition promised in their highly processed forms. If you are dairy tolerant, use a small amount of the highest quality dairy only. If you are not dairy tolerant there are wonderful delicious options, but they need to be fresh, not processed. Learn to make fresh nut milk easily from the simple recipe provided on page 44 (in the recipe section).

Infant Formula

Many families are at some point faced with choosing an infant formula. Improvements have been made in organic formulas including in some cases the elimination of palm oil, of the preservative palmitate, of solvent extracted DHA and the reduction of arsenic levels that were due to brown rice sweeteners. The choice of sweetener continues to be a primary concern and ranges from partially hydrolized corn based maltodextrin to organic sugar and brown rice syrup. Several formula brands also contain carageenan, a food additive that promotes inflammation in the body. Carageenan is used to stabilize an emulsion so that it won't separate. It is used in many dairy products. The synthetic preservatives ascorbyl palmitate and synthetic betacarotene are currently included in all the organic baby formulas except Baby's Only Organic by Natures One. This is frequently the best choice of formula and reads about +5.3. Parents Choice Organic, Similac Organic and Whole Foods brand 365 Organic all read about the same (+4.3). Three other formula options, Bright Beginnings, Vermont Organics and Earth's Best Organic also all read about the same quality (+3.4).

Wheat, Grains And Gluten - Free

Fifty years ago the meaning of gluten free was not something one had to be concerned about unless there was something wrong with you, something fairly uncommon called celiac disease. Today tens of millions of Americans suspect they are having a bad reaction to wheat products and notice that they feel better if they don't eat those foods for awhile. That sensitivity to wheat products is not celiac disease and therefore gluten free is not the whole answer. There are many reasons for adverse reactions to products made with processed grains, including many which are gluten free.

Reaction to the glyphosate signature on genetically modified wheat, corn and soy causes the most serious problems for most people. Glyphosate may be present in the flour, in the oil and the sweetener in many products. In addition to this primary chemical burden there are preservatives, flour conditioners called bromating agents, artificial colors and flavors and chemical sweeteners. Americans are embracing a wheat free, gluten free diet at a rate that vastly exceeds by tens of millions, the number of celiac cases. Wheat free and grain free is not a fad. It is a reaction to adulterated food products that make people increasingly unhealthy and it's a trend that's here to stay. However, changing to gluten-free and still eating a diet that is 30% or more grain based (remember grain, oils and grain sweeteners count too) and a diet that is largely composed of processed convenience foods will not create or restore health because it will not support healthy blood glucose levels or normal pH and hydration. Processed grains are dehydrating and acidifying and in many cases their nutritional quality is compromised, particularly in products with the longest shelf life.

To solve the health problems caused by over consumption of highly refined and chemically toxic grain based foods such as breads, pasta, cereal, crackers, cookies, pretzels, and chips, we need to do several things. The first priority is to choose ultra fresh and make ultra fresh. Grind your own grains. The bags on the shelf in the store may be many months older than you think. It's best to make everything fresh, even pasta, and to use the very best ingredients. Nuts and oats are soft and are easy to grind fresh at home in a high powered blender. For other flours, whether wheat or gluten free, choose small bags and store them in the freezer. The oils in grains that are not fresh ground and stored cold will be rancid. Because using only fresh food eliminates so many convenient but unhealthy options, overall quantity of processed grains consumed will be greatly reduced. Less processed grains in the diet raises pH and improves hydration, and it may also significantly improve nutrition. Overfed and undernourished is the usual outcome of consuming too great a proportion of one's diet in the form of highly processed grains.

Using oils from nuts and seeds such as walnut oil and sunflower seed oil instead of grain oils made from corn, soy and canola will also provide a better balance of health and nutrition. Most people do well on a diet that contains about 10% grains. The modern American diet composed of highly refined convenience foods is often as much as 50% grain based (flours, oils and sweeteners), as well as nearly 50% non-nutritive. The most common mistake made in switching to a wheat free diet is failure to understand that bagels, bread, cereal and pasta are not very good for us and should be used more as treat food than as a dominant food group. We love the rich comfort of grain based foods, pancakes, waffles, cookies, scones, rolls, biscuits, muffins, cakes and pies, but our bodies do not run efficiently on these foods alone. The body needs healthy fats, healthy proteins and the nutrient rich enzyme packed advantage of fruits and vegetables.

Eating no processed grains at all does not diminish the nutritional quality of one's diet. Choosing gluten free toaster waffles over wheat toaster waffles is not the change required to create sustainable health. Choosing not to eat toaster waffles ever and only eating waffles made from scratch from fresh eggs, healthy oil, and maybe some almond flour in those gluten free grains, that is a choice that will keep you from eating waffles more often than is good for your health. Those homemade fresh waffles will not only be much better for you, but the fact that you don't have them as often is also much better for you. The objective of a healthy diet would not be to change out all the current wheat containing products for their identical but gluten free version. The objective is to eat ten percent or less of your diet from grain based sources and to use fresh healthier choices to make up that ten percent. Among the substitutes available to replace wheat in the diet are quinoa, bean flour (garbanzo, fava bean), oat flour, rice flour, potato flour, tapioca flour, sorghum and almond flour. Recently coconut flour has been added as well as coconut in many other forms. These flours do not contain gluten and they do not contain glyphosate.

Quinoa - however, is fifteen dollars a pound and when processed into flour it does not produce a nutritionally superior product. Quinoa flour generally reads zero, safe, neutral, but with such a high price tag, it is possible to make choices that are much more beneficial.

Rice flour - is low protein and high carbohydrate nutritionally and does not produce the desired lightness and texture for cakes, breads and cookies unless mixed with other gluten free flours.

Brown rice flour - products were recently found to contain high levels of arsenic because the outer husk on the rice functions to take up the toxins from the soil and water and concentrate them in the outer husk and not in the inner white portion of the rice grain. Science has finally proven that mankind has not been polishing rice for ten thousand years out of some form of misguided vanity. It was actually wisdom passed down for millennia that kept humanity producing high quality white rice by polishing off the outer husk which eliminated dangerous toxins that may be present in water and soil. Because the research on arsenic in brown rice products was widely published, many manufacturers have already changed their products to reduce the danger.

Sorghum, fava bean, garbanzo, oat and nut flours - Heavier flours like sorghum, fava bean, garbanzo, oat and nut flours are all excellent for pancakes, cookies, pizza dough and biscuits. Experimenting with mixing together several different gluten free flours usually produces the best results. Of all the gluten free options for baking, only fresh ground nuts gets a high positive reading. The other flour substitutes will generally read zero at best but can be used to make food of positive nutritional value by the addition of healthy oils, fruits, vegetables, eggs, nuts and spices.

Gluten free foods made with these various flours are very high on the glycemic index and metabolize as sugar. They rapidly raise blood glucose and insulin levels and increase risk for diabetes and heart disease. Nut flours add protein and healthy oils metabolize more slowly, producing less blood sugar rise.

Coconut flour - does not contribute positive nutritional support though it is widely advertised as nearly miraculous due to its high fiber and low glycemic index. In the readings for my clients, coconut flour consistently reads at -4 and rather than beneficial fiber, the coconut flour reads as harmful to the transverse and descending colon where it produces a sluggish bowel and delayed evacuation, exactly the opposite of advertising claims and the magazine articles that have come out in favor of the many new highly refined processed coconut products. The greatest weakness of the paleo-diet is its reliance on processed foods, including the recommendation of these refined coconut products.

Healthy Meat

I grew up in a ranching family. My granddad was a cattle rancher and my family tradition includes numerous songs that were sung to the cattle when keeping company with them at night. My mother was a rancher as well. She raised horses and pigs. There were five hundred enormous pigs at a time on her family ranch, complete with shade trees and sprinklers and kids riding piggy back for real. My family raised and ate healthy meat. Beef and pork that is raised in a natural environment have very different qualities and effect on the body than does the meat produced by industrial agriculture.

Natural meat that is not sick from being fed an unnatural GMO grain based diet can be important in a therapeutic diet where nutrient dense broth is recommended for rebuilding the digestive system by reducing the mass or amount of physical matter being processed. Fresh homemade broths quickly raise protein levels for rebuilding and regeneration while supporting optimal hydration. There are many plant based proteins which support optimal hydration as well, so those whose spiritual practice includes a vegan or vegetarian diet are not forced to change that in order to get well. It does, however, take a good deal more commitment, attention and care to maintain adequate levels of high quality proteins without the use of broth. Protein powders do not read as beneficial to the body and metabolize as more sugar than protein.

Meat that is produced by today's industrialized feed lot methods is not safe for human consumption. The overall general reading on this meat is -8. The animals are unhealthy at slaughter and mass production methods contaminate the meat with deadly e-coli bacteria. Industrialized meat production on a grand scale to feed hundreds of millions cheaply has produced an unhealthy product that disrupts fat metabolism, produces hormone imbalance and contains a toxic chemical residue that weakens the immune system and contributes to the development of heart disease and cancer. Grass fed beef is healthier than grain fed beef. Locally produced grass fed beef is a better choice than grass fed beef from Peru, previously frozen.

Seafood comes from the same waters that are devastated by the Gulf Oil Spill, the Fukashima radiation leak and multiple garbage gyres. To have healthy seafood we would have to restore healthy seas. Yes, there is still some safe seafood available, but the supply and the options are rapidly diminishing. Less safe sea food could quickly become no safe sea food if steps are not taken to restore the ocean eco-system, to reduce ocean acidification and to clean up the garbage. There are dead zones developing, particularly in coastal regions, where the ocean no longer is capable of supporting life. During episodes called red tide, ocean temperatures together with toxic waters, (usually from fertilizer run off) combine to create an environment that is lethal to multicellular organisms. Everything dies and the decaying bodies wash up on shore and the air becomes noxious until the red tide episode is over and the beaches are clean of rotting fish. Given these conditions, any fish that might read safe to eat as I write these words, may no longer be safe by the time they are published. Because of the potential for rapid change in what seafoods may not be safe to eat, I recommend checking with safefishlist.org for most current issues and answers.

FAKE FOOD   REAL POISON

The Food Is Fake.   The Poison Is Real.

The American food supply is laden with toxic chemicals that are banned in most of the world. These additives are used to produce and preserve colors, prevent mold and extend shelf life and to affect texture, volume and flavor of processed foods. These additives are highly profitable for manufacturers and they are in many cases known carcinogens and neurotoxins. Our government says we are getting safe acceptable levels of these chemicals. Scientists worldwide say that isn't so and many other national governments agree with their research and have declared these additives unsafe for consumption by their citizens.

Among the widely banned chemicals still allowed in American processed foods are the petroleum sourced artificial food dyes that are often used in desserts, cereals, and children's medications. The worst of all, according to my attunement, is Blue #1, followed closely by Red #2, Red #40, Yellow #5 & #6. These food dyes have been found to promote brain cancer, nerve and cell damage and hyperactivity.

The innocuous sounding bromenated vegetable oil, is actually a flame retardant used to make foam insulation. Called BVO, this additive is also used in sodas, sports drinks, peanut butter and many processed meats. BVO is known to promote birth defects, brain damage and some forms of mental illness when consumed. Three more additives in our foods that are recognized as dangerous are potassium bromate, propylene glycol and carageenan. Bromate is a flour conditioner and blocks iodine, thereby damaging the thyroid. Propylene glycol is a preservative chemically akin to anti-freeze. Carageenan is a stabilizer used to keep emulsions from separating. It is found in heavy cream, infant formulas and yogurts. It is a known inflammatory agent in the body and could be a promoter of arthritis, cancer and many other chronic degenerative diseases.

Sodium benzoate and potassium benzoate are both preservatives. They are frequently used to prevent mold in soda pop. These chemicals interact with the plastic of the bottles to produce benzene, a known carcinogen that particularly damages the thyroid.

Two other common preservatives, BHT and BHA, are also proven carcinogens known to promote tumor growth. Preservatives in processed meats, sodium nitrate and sodium nitrite, have proven particularly destructive to the liver and pancreas. They are both on the list of known and widely banned carcinogens.

Aluminum, which is considered a toxic heavy metal when ingested, is an ingredient in non-dairy creamers, processed cheeses, baking mixes and infant formula. It is also prevalent in pesticides, antiperspirants and medications. Aluminum is known to promote brain damage leading to memory loss and dementia. Almost half the aluminum being consumed in America today may be from aluminum drink cans which leach aluminum molecules into the acidic beverage they so conveniently contain.

Monosodium glutamate, also called MSG and autolyzed or hydrolized yeast extract, is a chemical food additive that effects human brain chemistry, both in that it is a neuro-excitatory stimulant and in its intended effect to convince the brain that the food tastes better than it actually does. When fast food and processed foods taste better than they should and when food of poor quality tastes great, it is the magic of MSG. This food additive can cause nausea, headache, vomiting and restless agitation. It can also get you to eat food that doesn't really feed you but only makes you hungry for more, while leaving you depleted of energy and generally unwell.

Fast foods are frequently loaded with many dangerous food additives, but the petroleum derived preservative used in producing french fries is also known specifically for producing stomach tumors. This chemical preservative, TBHQ, can and should be eliminated, but remember doing so only partly redeems our beloved fries because high temperature deep fat frying produces hydrogenated oils. Hydrogenated oils have been changed biochemically in molecular structure by the high temperature and are particularly damaging to the liver, gall bladder and heart. One more possible ingredient in those already perilous french fries is the silicone based anti-foaming agent dimethyl polysiloxane. It's also used to make silly putty and caulk. Somewhere along the line, this product sold as fast food french fries, stopped being food.

Partially hydrogenated soy bean oil and cotton seed oil contribute more than one problem to the food supply. Currently called trans fats, hydrogenated oils disrupt normal lipid metabolism in the body and promote obesity, liver weakness and clogged arteries. The second toxic contribution from these oils is the herbicide glyphosate. This chemical is accurately classified as a biocide. Which is to say, destructive to all life. French research published in 2009 concluded that glyphosate kills human placental cells and produces infertility.

Much of America's food supply is contaminated with this toxic chemical. The cheap industrial foods designed to provide processed convenience foods to the masses at less than the price of whole fresh food are most often manufactured from one or more of the subsidized GMO crops.

These are crops that have been genetically modified such that the plants can be sprayed with the chemical herbicide and not die, though the plants around them which are not modified to withstand the poison will die. The modified plants take the chemical from the soil and water into its cells and there it remains until it is fed to livestock or processed into HFCS or other industrial food products. The full effects of glyphosate on other living organisms, especially those not genetically designed to withstand its deleterious effects are not yet known, but primary concerns are its effect on reproductive health and its role in the gradual loss of cognitive function and development of dementias. There is a price for the miracle of texture, taste and conveniently long shelf life (at home as well as from production to time of purchase) and that price is not the cash paid for the product. The price is malnutrition and obesity in the same body. The price is a debt the body pays in the form of disease and disability.

We want the convenience of food that lasts for months, in warehouses, on store shelves and in home pantries and refrigerators. We have an aging food supply and our continued use of those food products that are one to two years old at the time of consumption means a continuing dependance upon the chemical preservatives and additives that are used to manufacture them. However, manufacturers who use these methods to produce food for sale in America have responded to the demands of the world market and removed these dangerous additives from products produced for the European markets or Japan. Our government has not required that products be made equally safe if they are manufactured for sale to Americans, (as yet), nor have we as a people insisted upon it.

"It would be worthwhile to look again at the most basic key to our continuing good health: the food we eat".

Yogi Bhjan

LEARNING FROM EXPERIENCE

With the advent of the industrial age, the basic nature and quality of the modern diet changed very rapidly. The pre-industrial diet metabolized at a lower glucose level and produced lower insulin levels than the food of today. Food source and processing has changed the micro and macronutrient composition of food as well as its acid alkaline balance and its essential fatty acid content. Sodium-potassium ratios differ greatly in processed food (high sodium) compared to whole food which has higher potassium. This affects osmotic pressures and assimilation efficiency as well as effective elimination of waste, particularly micro waste. The larger issue of elimination of waste is the lack of natural fiber in the highly refined convenience foods as compared to whole foods and the resultant loss of both bowel health and general health due to sluggish elimination and constipation.

More significant than all of these changes combined is the chemical burden of herbicides, insecticides, preservatives and artificial colors, flavors, emulsifiers and even the packaging of convenience foods such as aluminum cans or BPA in plastics. The human body is a chemical factory and different organs and systems rely on different chemistry to regulate their functions. The chemicals in the food supply disrupt the normal chemistry of the body's operating systems and replaces them with messages that initiate destructive processes or promote the further deterioration of advancing disease.

Whole grains have long been promoted as part of a healthy diet, but the very meaning of the words has changed in just the last few years. Not long ago, grain that was ground for processed food was called whole grain if nothing was substantially removed by or in the milling process; for instance brown bread instead of white bread was more whole grain. Today whole grain needs to mean that these grains were not ground months ago to produce flours, oils and sweeteners that have been deteriorating in nutritional quality ever since and going rancid. Whole grains, if we mean it to be healthy, means things that are whole when you start, and if they are to be ground, then they are ground fresh. Whole grain needs to mean grain that contains the full nutritional value without the added chemical burden. GMO grains should not qualify for the label whole grain because they have been so significantly altered as to change their effect in the body due to the action of the chemicals on human physiology.

Each era has had its challenges to human health: plagues, famines, droughts and pestilence. Food adulteration, both through ignorance and through fraud, has been part of the challenge to human welfare for as long as there has been poverty and starvation. Famine foods, those non-food items that are substituted for food that is not available during times of war or natural disaster, are harmful to health and may simply change the cause of death from starvation to poisoning. In addition to those dangerous non-food items that are consumed to ease real starvation, there is also the entertainment category of non-food or fake food consumption. The consumer knows it's not food and doesn't care, but would like to be safe in consuming their favorite confection or snack.

Over one hundred fifty years ago our ancestors were learning that their food contained many dangerous substances that were there to improve taste, appearance and marketability and to retard or even hide spoilage. Oxide of lead was in wide spread use because it tasted deliciously sweet, improving the flavor of wines and candies and also providing a red coloring. Copper was used to make pickles the desirable green color the customers preferred and to color candies as well. Sulphuric acid was used in making vinegar. Alum was used for bleaching flour to make cheaper quality grains produce a product with the appearance of one made from higher quality grains. Alum is a double sulfate made of aluminum sulfate combined with another, either potassium sulfate or sodium sulfate. Alum causes digestive pain, cramping and diarrhea even in very small amounts. The market place had a demand for these food products but the consumer was being unknowingly harmed until scientists began testing foods that came under suspicion for harmful ingredients.

Many dangerous toxins have been eliminated from the food supply and from the water supply in the last two centuries. Many new dangers and toxins have entered the food and water supplies in the last forty years that will prove to be the source or primary cause of many modern epidemics including diabetes, cancer and Alzheimer's. Taking responsibility for safely feeding billions of people is a big job. It is inevitable that some glitches would appear as we work through the process. We are human, which means we are brilliant but limited beings who don't have all the details worked out yet. We are learning not to consume toxins but other motives (including convenience, profit and social acceptance) can all contribute their influence to episodes of not avoiding known problem foods and non-food consumables.

The challenges to our health and wellness today are different than they have been in the past. Both the internal environment of the human body and its external environment provide an array of challenges that are significantly different than those faced by our ancestors. For instance, in the area of vaccination, it is clear that there has been an abundance of good done by judicious use of vaccines for centuries. However, when the vaccination modality of disease prevention was first applied successfully, there were no toxic adjudavants (preservatives) in the prepared vaccine. Today's vaccines, given in ever increasing numbers, contain known neurotoxins such as mercury or aluminum as preservatives.

The Hepatitis B vaccine, which is given at birth, 3 months and 6 months is adjudavated with aluminum. Widely published research on the laboratory findings on this vaccine reveals that it is known to damage liver cells and that it is routinely being given to the most vulnerable population, newborns. Scientists believe the preservative used in the manufacture of the vaccine may be the promoter of the development of liver weakness or liver disease. When vaccines were still a safe natural therapy, they were prepared fresh without any preservative. But this safer way of preparing vaccines does not generate billion dollar profits. This debate needs to end. It is not vaccine theory that is at fault. It is the vaccines themselves, that by their formulation, ingredients, manufacturing processes, storage conditions and parameters of administration, are causing harm and controversy. The newborn immune system is immature and yet it is bombarded with about twenty-four doses of vaccine toxins in the first 24 months of life.

Some children's constitutions bear the onslaught of this unnatural challenge better than others. For some, recovery from over immunization and vaccine damage can take years. For others, full recovery never happens and families are left with confusion about how to make the best choices. In this country, vaccination is the law unless an exemption is granted. It may be an unjust law. It may be misguided. The decision to inject neurotoxins and poisonous chemicals along with the vaccine is certainly worthy of deepest careful consideration. It may even be worthy of civil disobedience or non-violent non-co-operation in our best Ghandiesque style to change what needs to change to protect the best interests of humanity, not just collectively but individually as well. Avoiding all toxins is impossible in modern life. Avoiding all the toxic choices you can is still wisely guided.

"To a significant degree, we are an overfed and undernourished nation digging an early grave with our teeth, and lacking the energy that could be ours because we overindulge in junk foods".

Ezra Taft Benson

Super food is one of the current popular labels meant to indicate the most nutrient dense and bioavailable foods to support health and wellbeing. Many foods which are widely marketed as nutritional powerhouses are not only not beneficial, they are frequently harmful to many who are persuaded by the propaganda of the marketplace.

SUPER FOODS AND NOT SO SUPER

Manuka honey: +3.6 (if used raw, zero, neutral when cooked)
Other raw honey: +3 (if used raw, zero, neutral when cooked)
Bee Pollen: zero
Royal jelly: zero
Maple syrup: zero to +4
Maca powder - raw, adaptogen, liver & adrenal support: +4.2
Cacao powder - raw, if used raw: zero
Kombucha - commercially processed: -4.2
        bottled: -4.3,
        homemade fresh: zero
reads: +4.3 for diarrhea
Pomegranate: +9.2 fresh (bottled pomegranate juice: zero)
Coconut water - commercially processed: -3.2
        fresh, whole green & brown - water & flesh: zero nutritively
        reads: +4.2 for hydration
Coconut oil - raw: -4.2
        cooked: -8.2
        topically: +4.2
Protein powders: -3.2 (even the raw ones)
Green powders: zero
        spirulina: zero
        blue green algae: zero
Raw almonds, soaked: +9.3 almond cream, almond milk & dressings
Walnuts, raw: +8.5
Pecans, raw: +7.9
Seeds, raw sunflower & pumpkin: +9.4
Cashews, raw soaked & cashew cream: +8.3
Cashews, raw un-soaked: +8.4
Chia seed: -3.2,
Hemp seed: zero
Processed hemp milk: -9.2
Processed soy milk: -5.2
Processed rice milk: -5.2

Processed almond milk: -8.2
Sprouts - sunflower: +9.2
       micro-greens: +9.8
Spinach, raw: +9.2
Watercress: +9.2
Cilantro: +7.4
Basil: +6.4
Kale: +1.2
Chard: zero
Raw juice: +9.4 to 9.8
Broth, homemade, grass fed beef: +8.4
Organic chicken broth: +7.2
Bone broth: +9.4
Fish broth: +8.4
Veggie broth: +3.2
Raw oils - walnut (for salad): +9.2
       olive: +8.4
       sunflower: +9.3
       organic butter: zero
       ghee: zero
       canola oil: -4.3

"Doctors of the future will have less use of medicines of any kind. Instead, they will instruct patients in the correct ways of eating, proper care of the human frame, and the right attitude that facilitates healing of both the mind and the body."

Thomas Edison

UNIVERSAL PROTOCOL FOR SUSTAINABLE HEALTH

1. Keep hydration in optimal range by using structured water daily. Raw juice 2 to 3 cups daily, high protein broth, avoid grains and processed foods.

2. Keep pH in optimal range: raw food raises pH, cooked food lowers pH, processed foods lower pH, stress and high cortisol lower pH, high protein lower cortisol and supports raising pH, optimal hydration raises pH, drugs, alcohol and prescription medications lower pH.

3. Diet - balance of 30 to 32% of assimilatable proteins and less than 15% sugar, avoid grains and processed foods (many of which metabolize as sugars), avoid GMO's, glyphosate is a cumulative toxin, avoid industrial dairy, use organic only, avoid industrial meats, use natural and grass fed. No microwave.

4. Exercise - 60 minutes daily, especially include walking, stretching, balance, resistance bands, biking, hula hoops, skating, dancing, yoga. Focus on core strength, flexibility and stamina. Must be fun.

5. Supplements - a healthy person on a healthy diet does not need vitamins and supplements.

Vitamin A - nutritionally sourced, carrot juice.

Vitamin B - B100 complex daily for most people. Up to 2 x day under extreme stress (discontinue when stress level is down to 3.4.).

Vitamin C - 3x day, 2 grams per dose x 3 weeks for any acute immune challenge. For 3 to 4 months for chronic challenge and adrenal support.

Vitamin D - regulated through proper pH and mineral balance, natural sunlight and Reuteri.

Vitamin E - Indications for supplementation are diminished cognitive health / brain function and heart health including atherosclerosis. Use pure d-alpha tocopherol only, not mixed tocopherols, 800 I.U.'s daily.

CoQ10 - indications for CoQ10 include chronic high stress / cortisol flooding, cognitive decline, poor physical fitness, heart health, exhaustion, migraines. Use 300 to 400 mgs 2 x day.

Magnesium - indications: chronic anxiety, worry, stress, insomnia, constipation, food and leg cramps. Natural Calm.

Calcium - indications: acidosis, thyroid weakness, osteoporosis and all recovery of bone and dental health. 1 gram 2 x day, coral calcium or raw calcium.

Iron - indications: anemia, malnutrition, pregnancy. Use liquid Floradix Floravital, gluten free.

Zinc - indications: pituitary (hormone), prostate.

Selenium - indications: cancer.

Potassium - nutritionally sourced, all raw food is full of potassium.

ProGest progesterone cream - insomnia, bones, vein walls, skin.

Alpha lipoic acid - brain, liver, fat metabolism.

Reuteri - colon health, chelates out yeast, arsenic and glyphosate.

Digestive Enzymes - indications: stomach bloat, gas, constipation or sluggish bowels.

Quercetin - indications: allergies, hives, rash, itching, watery eyes, hyperimmune and autoimmune response.

Flor-Essence - gentle liquid herbal detox formula.

Oregano oil - suppressed infection, teeth, nail fungus, pneumonia.

GSE - grapefruit seed extract, tooth and gum infection, nail fungus, colds and flu.

6. Therapeutic modalities - Castor oil packs, cranial/sacral adjustments, massage, emotional release work, LED light therapy (blue)

7. Psychological health and happiness - stress, rest, balance, observing 'alarmist' thinking and critical outlook, intentional resilience, confidence, optimism, enthusiasm, meditation, prayer, chanting, music, journaling, Sabbath, effortless being

8. Sleep - rest, naps, solitude, quiet time

9. Meaningful work, right livelihood, service

10. Home health / First aid supplies - GSE (grapefruit seed extract), iodine, jojoba oil & carrot seed oil, hypericum, Colon Clenz, calendula ointment, Traumeel, Epsom salts, salt, SsstingStop, aloe vera gel, Rescue Remedy, Beret Jane Miracle Salve, castor oil, heating pad

FOOD POWER: 12 WEEKS TO SUSTAINABLE HEALTH

Because the idea of doing a total make over on one's diet is intimidating due to the scope and detail the undertaking requires of us, it may be more approachable when broken down into short term goals and priorities. The steps outlined below can be done in almost any order and at any pace. Each change could be added at a two week interval, or a 10 day interval or any other customized schedule that seems to best fit your personal needs. This process of adding in specific healthy choices and eliminating a related unhealthy choice at the same time moves one steadily towards the goal of a holistic natural and healthy pattern of eating that optimizes the body's ability to heal.

<u>Add Healthy</u> and	<u>Let Go of Unhealthy</u>
week 1. **Raw juice** - 3 cups = 30% raw food diet. Carrots, blueberries, spinach, red grapes (3 recipes on pg. 38-39)	Wheat
week 2. **Broth** - bone broth, fish, beef & chicken (2 recipes on pg. 49-50)	Soy
week 3. **Soaked Raw Nuts** - almond cream almond milk, dressings (5 recipes on pg. 42, 43, 46, 47)	HFCS & aspartame/ Nutrasweet
week 4. Healthy Proteins - all natural meats and fish	Non-Organic dairy

week 5. **Healthy Oils** - sunflower, safflower, walnut and olive oils

Chocolate

week 6. **Healthy Snacks** - more nuts and seeds raw walnuts, cashews, pecans, sunflower, and pumpkin seeds.

Fried Foods

week 7. **Sprouts & Micro-greens** - (4 recipes on pg. 40, 41)

Microwave

week 8. **Homemade Salad Dressing** (5 recipes on pg. 42, 43)

Prepared frozen dinners, meals and frozen desserts. Convenience foods

week 9. **Healthy dessert** - bliss balls, dried fruits and raw pies (see recipes on pg. 43-48)

Unhealthy oils, Canola oil, cottonseed oil, soy bean oil, GMO corn oil

week 10. **Healthy beverage** - agua fresca's, fruit waters-lemon/lime/orange,ginger tea (3 recipes on pg. 50, 51)

Protein Powder

week 11. **Healthy food balance** – add 60% raw food diet, use organic only

GMO potatoes

week 12. **Healthy salt** - pink, celtic sea salts

Candy, commercial

If you also want your new habits to support weight loss, do your exercise in the morning before you eat (4 oz. juice if you need something) and do not eat after 9 pm. To regulate your sleep, also exercise at the beginning of your day, ideally about 8 am.

A friend of mine and a very inspired intuitive healer in her own right, mentioned to me that people can't realistically make all the changes I recommended at one time. She suggested dividing the recommended changes up into a series of steps that people could take in a specific order that would provide a better support system for accomplishing the larger goal of sustainable health. Each step very specifically provides one or more of these 4 essentials: healthy fats, (EFA's) essential fatty acids, pH, and hydration. These absolutely essential elements are exactly what's most often missing in the every day challenge of creating health, strength and wellness.

The instructions contained in this 12 week protocol for changing from unhealthy to healthy also contains an abundance of food sourced nutrients, vitamins and minerals. Recipes for making salads, salad dressings, desserts, snacks, nut milks, broths and raw juices are all included. If it is still too difficult to get exactly what you need to be eating because it needs to be fresh made, consider buying from a local raw food chef and from farmer's markets to get variety of sprouts, greens, raw honey and fresh eggs, as well as jams and pickles.

> **"Everything is energy and that's all there is to it. Match the frequency of the reality you want and you cannot help but get that reality. It can be no other way. This is not philosophy. This is physics".**
>
> **Albert Einstein**

RAW JUICE

For detoxing the body and recovery from long term chronic illness, raw juice is one of the most frequent recommendations that will be given. Daily raw fruit and vegetable juice is the fastest way to raise the pH to ideal levels and therefore supports kidney function to speed detoxing of the body. Daily raw juice is also the best support for healing the adrenals, recovery of vitality and anti-aging. Raw juice is the best source of progesterone for peri-menopausal and post-menopausal women, as well as an excellent support for weight loss and cognitive recovery or resilience.

The two basic types of juicing are extraction juicing, which separates out the pulp, and blended raw juice made from whole foods with all the natural fiber kept in the drink. The extraction juice is more nutrient dense and is specifically recommended for recovery from chronic illness or malnutrition. Blended whole juices are more fiber dense and more suitable for those who have greater health and digestive function to begin with. Blended juices are excellent for maintaining good health. Extraction juices are good for recovery or for maintenance of sustainable health. Extraction juicing makes it much easier to consume the 63 servings of raw fruits and vegetables per week that is recommended for a therapeutic diet intended to raise pH and increase hydration. Blended juices, with their high fiber content, in some cases, cause stomach bloating and discomfort, especially for those with significantly compromised digestion such as Leaky Gut Syndrome.

Frequently, the addition of raw nut cream to the raw juice is recommended to create a high protein drink that is a superfood for the brain. Rich in omega 3 essential fatty acids, raw almond cream also supports a leptin response from the brain indicating that it has been fed and satisfied and effectively turning off the appetite/hunger signal. The addition of the raw nut cream makes the raw juices much more palatable to children as it softens the taste, more like a cream soda, smooth and easy, tasty and delicious and one of the best possible food choices for the body. Do not use processed protein powders in your raw juices, even those that say raw. Even the very best of these is a highly refined processed food and will metabolize as 28% sugar or higher and only 20% protein.

It's important for beginners to not be overly challenged with the taste combinations of raw juice when they are first learning to juice. Make the combinations tasty and within the comfort zone of each individual with no more than 25% to 30% greens, especially for anyone feeling resistant to the experience. Simple combinations of familiar and well liked flavors will be most appealing. In the extraction juicer, run the greens through together with a juicier fruit at the same time, such as grapes or pears, to rinse the green juice through the sieve basket.

Is carrot juice and fruit juice too sweet? Unless you have a candida overgrowth, no it is not too sweet. It is, in most cases, what will work best to support a shift away from a diet that has been metabolizing at about 30% sugar due to consumption of a large percentage of processed foods, particularly grains. For those new to juicing, carrot juice and apple and spinach are common early favorites. Organic is always best but may not always be an option due to price or availability. Buy organic whenever possible but regular carrots from a grocery store is a better choice than no carrot juice at all and taking advantage of sale prices for local produce which is in season usually provides many delicious choices. Drink raw juice immediately. It will not keep very well for longer than two hours.

To estimate amounts, figure one large carrot per ounce or two small carrots. One medium large apple makes about two ounces of juice and two cups of loose greens produces about an ounce of green juice. Common choices of greens are spinach, watercress, cilantro and mint and sometimes basil. Kale is an option but is often not popular with beginners and children. Kale is not recommended for juice because it inhibits iodine assimilation.

The greens especially support detoxing and healing the liver and making healthy blood. Common fruit choices for raw juice include apples, pears, grapes, blueberries, strawberries or mixed berries, peaches, lemons, limes and kiwis. Most commonly juiced vegetables include carrots, the greens mentioned, tomatoes, cucumbers, celery, beets and ginger. Celery can cause stomach upset for some who may be sensitive. Use it only if it easily agrees. It has a slightly salty flavor which combines well with other vegetables. Beets have a strong musty taste, especially the beet greens, and should be used in small proportion. Ginger is also used only in very small amount, less than 1 teaspoon fresh grated ginger per 16 ounce juice (sometimes much less). Fresh ginger raises pH and helps heal the mucosal lining of the intestines.

A simple mix that makes 16 oz. and is palatable for most beginners: 7 oz. carrot juice, 5 oz. apple juice and 4 oz. spinach. Add 2 tablespoons high protein raw almond cream to create a smoothie.

Also popular is: 6 oz. carrot juice, 8 oz. orange juice and 2 oz. pineapple juice or strawberry juice. Again, add 2 tablespoons raw almond cream to make a high protein smoothie with a gentler taste.

Baby food: age 18 months and up: plain carrot juice, 2 oz. or carrot juice with raw almond cream

Afternoon juice: 11 oz. fresh raw tomato juice, 6 oz. cucumber juice, 1 oz. cilantro juice and 1/2 lime.

MAKING FOOD THAT HEALS

Barley Oat Sun Crisps (Raw Crackers)

1 cup barley, soaked 24 hours
2 cups thick cut oats, soaked for 6 hours
1 cup sunflower seeds, soaked for 6 hours
1 carrot, grated
pink Himalyan salt
fresh ground pepper
Blend in Vitamix for 3 min on low
Drop by spoonfuls on to parchment paper and press flat, thin
Dehydrate 8 to 10 hours

Sweet Potato Chips

Peel 1 yam, then slice thin with potato peeler
Apply pink Himalyan salt
Dehydrate 8 to 10 hours

Tomato Cucumber Avocado Salad

garden fresh tomatoes, slice thin and cut bite size
cucumber, peeled and sliced thin
scallions, sliced thin
cilantro, fresh whole leaves, torn individually
avocados, cubed
fresh lime juice
fresh minced garlic
pink Himalayan salt

fresh ground pepper
Serve over a bed of sunflower sprouts or water cress
Variation: add diced jicama

Large Spinach Salad

makes 6 + cups = to 2 salad meals or 6 side salads
3 cups fresh washed organic spinach
1 cup micro-greens or sunflower sprouts
2 cups fresh washed organic butter lettuce
organic red grapes - washed and cut in half, 1 to 2 cups
1 organic apple, diced
3/4 cup dried tart Montmorency cherries (Trader Joe's)
1 cup raw pecan pieces (or walnuts)
Feta cheese
Serve with lemon and oil dressing (or vinegar and oil)
Variations: add muddled (smashed) raspberries to lemon and oil dressing or change apple to diced organic pear and add pear to the lemon and oil dressing. Blend dressing and pear at high speed for 2 minutes. Use a soft ripe pear for this dressing so that it will blend to a creamy texture.

Lively Luncheon Salad

large, 6 + cups = 2 salad meals or 6 side salads
3 cups fresh washed organic romaine lettuce
2 cups butter lettuce or red leaf lettuce
1 cup fresh water cress
1 cup micro-greens or 1 cup sunflower sprouts or other sprouts
1 cup grated organic carrots
1 cup red grapes, cut in half
6 scallions (green onions) sliced thin, including greens
1 organic apple diced
2 large stalks of celery, de-stringed and diced or substitute
3/4 cup jicama, peeled and diced.
3/4 cup raw sunflower seeds (without shells) or substitute equal amount of raw pecan pieces

Cashew Lemon Dressing

1 & 1/2 cups raw cashews, soaked 24 hours (makes about 3 cups)
1/3 cup fresh lemon juice
1 teaspoon salt
1 teaspoon garlic powder or fresh pressed garlic
1/2 teaspoon each of dried basil & oregano, crushed
Add 1/2 cup pure water
Blend in Vitamix until smooth (3 minutes) adding more water as needed

Lemon & Oil Salad Dressing

1/2 cup fresh squeezed lemon or lime juice - limes are easier because they are not full of seeds
1/2 cup sunflower oil (or safflower) olive oil and walnut oil change the taste significantly
3/4 teaspoon sea salt or pink Himalayan salt
1/2 teaspoon dry oregano, rub between palms to crush fine
1/2 teaspoon dry basil, rub between palms to crush fine
3/4 teaspoon fine garlic powder or fresh pressed garlic
1/3 teaspoon fresh cracked pepper

Combine in a bottle and shake until well blended. The recipe is very flexible and amounts of lemon, oil and spices can vary according to personal taste. Most important is the ratio of salt to the lemon and oil mixture because salt is the only yang element in this otherwise very yin combination. When the balance of yin yang is achieved the dressing tastes perfect.

Option: this recipe can be adapted by the addition of 1/2 teaspoon dry mustard powder. Either version of this dressing is great for making potato salad. To 3 cups of cooked diced potatoes and 1 cup of diced celery and 2 hard boiled eggs diced add 1/2 cup of the lemon oil dressing or the lemon oil mustard dressing. Optional addition of 1/3 cup mayonnaise to make creamy potato salad.

Cilantro Lime Dressing

1 fresh bunch cilantro, about 3 cups
1/2 cup fresh lime juice
2 cups sunflower seeds, soaked 24 hours (makes about 4 cups)
1 teaspoon garlic powder or fresh pressed garlic
1 teaspoon salt
Add 3/4 cup pure water

Blend in Vitamix until smooth (3 minutes) adding more water if needed.

Fresh Tomato Salsa

5 or 6 organic tomatoes, diced (cut small)
3/4 of 1 sweet onion, diced fine
5 cloves of fresh garlic, diced fine or pressed
2 oz. diced fresh cilantro, about 4 tablespoons
1 can whole roasted green chiles (do not buy diced, cut them yourself).
1 1/2 to 2 teaspoons salt
Juice of 1 to 2 fresh limes, 3 to 4 tablespoons
For hotter salsa add fresh diced jalapeno, 1 to 2 teaspoons
Makes 5 to 6 cups.
Store in a glass container.

Refrigerator Pickles

Easy fresh homemade pickles. Absolutely the best.
Pickling cucumbers, smaller than standard
4 to 6 may be enough for 4 pint jars
A quick small batch of pickles in a variety of flavors.
Slice cucumbers
Onion - about 3/4 of 1 standard sweet onion, cut large
Pack onions and sliced cucumbers tightly into jars Add: 1/4 teaspoon dill
Variations: cilantro and red peppers or garlic cloves
In a pan, heat to boiling:
2 cups red wine vinegar (or garlic wine vinegar)
2 cups sugar
1/4 cup canning and pickling salt (non-Iodized)
2 teaspoons mustard seed
1/2 teaspoon tumeric
Remove from heat and allow to cool about 5 to 10 minutes. Pour hot mixture into jars over cucumbers and onions. Seal and refrigerate. Excellent for up to 10 months.

Almond Delight Fruit Pie

pie crust

2 cups almonds, ground fine (can use almond flour)
2 cups dates
2 cups dried apricots (I also put these through the grinder)
Blend in Vitamix until crumbly
Press into pie pans (forming edges first before bottom), makes 2 crusts

pie filling

2 cups almonds, soaked 24 hours, remove hulls (makes about 4 cups)
1 cup sunflower seeds, soaked
1 cup raisins, soaked (barely cover w/ water and include the water)
1/2 cup fresh honey comb (more if you prefer)
3 fresh apricots and 1 peach or 2 pears
1 teaspoon vanilla
Blend all in Vitamix for 3 minutes or until smooth and creamy
Add 3 tablespoons maca (optional superfood)
makes 2 pies
Pour a layer of fresh blueberries over bottom of pie crusts
Pour prepared filling into prepared pie crusts over blueberries
Chill for several hours or overnight and top with fresh strawberries, blueberries and fresh apricots, sliced thin and arranged artfully before serving

Bliss Balls - 4 Variations Of Raw Dessert

spice cake bites

1 cup almonds, ground fine
1 cup currants
1 cup of pecans, ground course
1 cup chopped medjool dates (about 12)
2 tablespoons honeycomb
2 tablespoons maca powder (optional)
1/2 teaspoon each of salt, cardamon, nutmeg
1 teaspoon cinnamon
Mix all ingredients together by hand and roll into small balls makes 24 to 30
Alternate version: for Persian style raw baklava bites use pistachio nuts instead of pecans

Bhakti Bliss Bites

1 cup almonds, ground fine
1 cup walnuts, ground course
1/2 cup sunflower seeds, ground course
1/2 cup pumpkin seeds, ground course
3/4 cup apricots, ground
1/2 cup medjool dates chopped
2 tablespoons honey comb
2 tablespoons maca powder (optional)
salt and cinnamon
Mix all ingredients together by hand and roll into small balls

Fruit Cake Bites

1 cup almonds, ground fine
1 cup walnuts, ground course
2 tablespoons maca powder
1/2 cup dried pineapple, ground
1/4 cup crystalized ginger, ground
1/2 cup medjool dates, chopped
2 tablespoons honeycomb
1/2 tsp each of salt, nutmeg, cloves
Mix together by hand and roll into small balls

Walnut Brownie Bites

1 cup raw almonds, ground fine
1 cup walnuts, ground course
1/2 cup raw cocoa powder
2 tablespoons maca powder (optional)
3 tablespoons honeycomb
1 cup medjool dates, chopped (about 12)
1/2 tsp salt
Mix together by hand and roll into small balls
Variation: add dry cherries, diced, for chocolate cherry bites

An assortment of any 2 or 3 raw dessert balls makes a fabulous dessert

Very Cherry Ensemble - Raw Food Pie

pie crust

2 cups raw pecans
1 cup medjool dates, chopped or ground
1 cup dried apricots, ground
1/2 teaspoon cinnamon
1/3 teaspoon cardamom
1/3 teaspoon nutmeg
Blend together in a Vitamix and press into a pie pan.
(optional - sun bake 2 hours) chill.

pie filling

1 cup raw, soaked, hulled almonds
1/2 cup soak water from dates
6 soaked medjool dates
1/2 cup crystalizing honey or honey comb
1 teaspoon natural vanilla
1/2 teaspoon cinnamon
1/2 teaspoon cardamom
1/3 teaspoon nutmeg
3/4 cup dried apricots, ground
Blend in a Vitamix until creamy. Add water or agave as needed. Spread 2 cups of sweet raw cherries over the filling and then cover with topping below.

topping

2 cups raw soaked cashews
1 cup soak water from dates
6 medjool dates, soaked
agave syrup as needed
1 teaspoon natural vanilla
Blend in Vitamix until light and fluffy. Set aside 1/2 of the cashew whip for later use.
Add 3 tablespoons of the filling mix to the remaining cup of cashew whip and blend.
Assemble - fill chilled crust with 2 cups fresh sweet raw cherries, cut in half (pitted), pour filling mix over cherries and smooth to edges. Top with a layer of cashew whip blended with the filling and add a few sliced cherries and sliced almonds on top in a decorative design. Serve with the extra cashew whip as desired.
Variations: use blueberries, blackberries or a berry assortment for the fresh fruit layer. Serve cold.

MJ's 1st Birthday Cake

2 cups raw almonds ground fine, sifted
Mix all dry ingredients together in a small bowl.
1 cup rice flour
2 teaspoons baking soda
1/2 teaspoon cinnamon
4 tablespoons meringue powder (or 3 egg whites)
3/4 cup raw agave syrup
1 1/2 cups natural applesauce
In a large mixing bowl, whip 4 tablespoons meringue powder with 4 tablespoons water to form stiff peaks (or use 3 egg whites)
While blending at medium speed, slowly add 3/4 cup raw agave syrup to stiff egg whites
Next, in the same way, slowly add 1 1/2 cups natural applesauce
Now add dry ingredients 1 cup at a time and blend until thoroughly mixed
Bake until toothpick inserted in center comes out clean (about 45 minutes for 9" pans)
Wheat free, oil free, sugar free, egg safe

Almond Cream

Soak 1 1/2 cups raw almonds for 36 hours, rinsing every 12 hours like sprouts
Pour into large bowl in clean water and remove the husks
The soaked almonds can be used immediately or stored in the refrigerator for later
Blend (in a Vitamix or Blendtec) the soaked almonds together with 1 cup of date water (4 to 6 large dates soaked in water for 2 to 12 hours) or substitute up to 3 tablespoons raw agave for dates, 1 teaspoon natural vanilla. Blend until smooth and creamy, adding more water as necessary to achieve desired consistency, varies to thick like hummus or light like whipped cream.
Add 2 tablespoons of raw almond cream to each glass of raw juice or use as dressing for Waldorf salad or as a dip for apple slices.
It will keep for up to a week in the refrigerator.

Almond cream is very high in Omega 3's and 6's and protein (28%) and supports production of the hormone Leptin in the brain

Almond Milk

Almond milk is the same recipe as almond cream but with the addition of a lot more structured water. The recipe above will make about 6 cups of almond milk. Pour it through a fine mesh bag to filter out the grainy texture from tiny fragments of nuts.

Pumpkin Fruit And Nut Cookies - Gluten Free

1 cup butter, softened to room temperature (2 sticks)
2 eggs (large organic cage free)
1 teaspoon vanilla
1 cup of brown sugar
Beat all together in a large bowl with an electric mixer on medium speed.
Next mix in 1 cup pumpkin (1 small can is 2 cups)
Separately combine dry ingredients in a bowl:
2 cups ground almond flour with 2 cups of Bob's Red Mill gluten free All Purpose Baking Flour*
tapioca flour, almond flour, buckwheat flour and rice flour
1 teaspoon salt
1 teaspoon baking powder
1 1/2 teaspoons baking soda
2 teaspoons cinnamon
1 teaspoon cardamon
1 teaspoon nutmeg

Add all dry ingredients, 1 cup at a time to the pumpkin, butter and egg mixture, and mix well.
Add: 3 cups dry fruit, cut small - currants, cherries, dates, dried pineapple, candied ginger, dried apricots.
1 cup raw sunflower seeds (and pumpkin seeds if desired).
1 cup raw pecan pieces or walnuts and mix well.
Refrigerate dough 2 hours or more.
Separate into portions and place on wax paper and roll up into a long tube for slicing.
Place slices on a greased cookie sheet and bake at 350 degrees for 15 minutes.
Store cookie dough rolls in freezer and use for small batches for fresh slice and bake comfort food.
Variation: This dough also works well for Thumbprint Cookies. Use soft dough, not frozen, and make an indentation in the middle of each cookie and fill with raspberry jam or orange marmalade.

*works well or make your own combination from 3 choices listed: 4 cups gluten free flours - can include oat flour, fava bean, garbanzo bean, potato flour, sorghum

BROTHS - BEEF, CHICKEN, BONE & MARROW BROTHS

Beef Broths

Place a portion of grass fed beef into crock pot. Use about 16 oz. of meat (including bones) to 8 cups of water. Add 1/2 onion, 3 or 4 garlic cloves, 2 to 3 carrots, Mushrooms can be added if desired. Cook about 12 hrs, salt & pepper to taste. Salt is very important in your broth as it is used by the body to make hydrochloric acid (HCL) in the stomach which breaks down food for digestion. Eating enough healthy salt also supports optimum hydration.

The nutritional value of the meat and vegetables is concentrated in the broth in a form that is easily assimilated by the body. The body can access proteins consumed as broth in as little as twenty minutes. Digesting whole flesh can take a couple of days. Using the nutrient dense broth, and not the solids, in this soup puts less burden on the body's digestive powers. The solids of meat and vegetables in the broth can be eaten for the comfort factor, the pure enjoyment, but one can also skip eating the solids for the broth and give them to someone else, a companion animal or even throw them away, in the interest of giving your digestive system the best support to speed healing both throughout the digestive system and throughout the body.

Chicken Broth

Option 1 - roast a whole all natural organic chicken and after serving the roast chicken as a meal, use the carcass, bones wings etc... to make soup stock. Using the roasted chicken gives the broth a richer, even perhaps sweeter flavor. Place the whole carcass or pieces in the crock pot and about 8 cups of water.

Also add: 1/2 onion, 3 to 4 garlic cloves, 2 to 3 carrots and 2 to 3 sticks of celery. The vegetables can be added whole and do not need to be cut up into pieces to make this kind of broth. For a southwestern flavor, hot chili peppers can also be added and just before serving, add a squeeze of fresh lime juice. Always salt and pepper to taste.

Option 2 - use pieces of uncooked natural organic chicken - perhaps a large breast piece or a few thighs. I do not make soup from chicken wings only. Place the raw chicken pieces in the crock pot and proceed as above allowing the stock to simmer for 10 to 12 hours.

Bone Broth

Use either one of the above recipes and strain out all of the content. What is left is pure bone broth. If one is truly ill this will be the easiest to digest, reserving energy for healing.

Nut Loaf

1 cups fresh shredded greens - spinach is best
2 tablespoons fresh herb - choose one (Basil, Cilantro or Parsley)
1 tablespoon fresh minced garlic
1 sweet medium onion, chopped fine
1 teaspoon dried oregano
1 teaspoon salt
Saute all in 2 tablespoons olive oil for 3 minutes, remove from heat, add 3 cups chopped nuts, blended crumbly but not flour, use walnuts, pecans or cashews.
Optional - 1 cup gluten free bread crumbs
Blend in 1 to 2 eggs, add 3 oz. tomato paste
Shape in a greased loaf pan and bake at 350 degrees for 45 to 50 minutes, cool 10 minutes before slicing.

Ginger Tea

3 inches of fresh ginger root, peeled and sliced, add 2 cups of water and bring to a boil, simmer for 10 to 15 minutes. Cool the ginger tea concentrate and add enough water to make 2 quarts of tea. Add fresh squeezed lime juice and agave or raw honey if desired. Makes a very light refreshing drink that can be enjoyed warm, cold or room temperature. Fresh homemade ginger tea heals the digestive track, supports the kidneys, raises pH and provides relief from aches and pains of arthritis and fibromyalgia. It is a healthy beverage for everyone and safe to consume 3 to 5 cups daily. If ginger tea burns the tongue like hot sauce then it is not diluted enough. Add additional water until it doesn't create any sensation of heat in the mouth.

Chai Tea

This is a traditional chai with both dairy and sweetener as well as caffeine from black tea.

In a large pot combine 4 to 5 cups of water, 10 to 12 whole cardamon seeds in shells, 2 cinnamon sticks, 6 to 8 whole cloves and 3/4 teaspoon of ground nutmeg.

Bring to a boil and simmer on low heat for 15 to 20 minutes. Remove from heat.

Add a strong black tea such as Sadaf with cardamon (from your middle-eastern market), English Breakfast tea or darjeeling.

Let steep for 5 minutes and remove tea leaves and loose spices with a strainer.

To 5 cups of tea add 2 cups of whole milk, half and half or 1 cup of whole cream and 1 cup of milk. Return to heat for 4 to 5 minutes to heat the milk but do not boil.

Add raw agave sweetener or honey to taste - approximately 1 teaspoon per cup.

Can be enjoyed hot or cold. This tea is renown for supporting a state of relaxed alertness.

Agua Frescas - Lightly Fruited Waters

The simplest version of an agua fresca is the now common practice of adding a slice of lemon to one's water. Just this one simple step alone is tremendously supportive to the kidneys. Raw fresh fruit in our water adds flavor, delight and health benefits of improved hydration and pH. Many fruits are very well suited for flavoring water including all citrus, pineapple, blueberries, raspberries, strawberries and pomegranate. Choose a pleasing combination of 2 to 3 fruits and mix about 15% to 20% fruits to 80% to 85% water. Serve lightly chilled.

Suggested combinations: cucumber, lime and mint leaves - orange slices, strawberries and pineapple - raspberries, pomegranate and lemon slices - strawberries, kiwi and mint leaves - raspberries, blueberries and blackberries

Healthy Spices

Natural spices contribute healing factors to many favorite recipes. For thousands of years, food and the spices used to prepare it have been treasured for their health benefits.

Cumin - curcumin, suppresses cancer cells

Turmeric - anti-aging, anti-inflammatory, brain health

Ginger - reduces inflammation throughout the body, anti-cancer, improves digestion, lowers blood pressure, improves bone health

Basil - supports liver detoxing and prevents blood clots, antioxidant

Oregano - anti-microbial(anti-infective) antiseptic and antioxidant

Garlic - supports lipid metabolism, heart health, healthy cholesterol, brain health

Rosemary - memory stimulant, recovery of brain health, antimicrobial

Cinnamon - calming yet alert, beneficial to brain and nerves, regulates blood sugar

Mint - improves digestion, supports liver, gall bladder, bile production

Mustard - anti-microbial, inhibits growth of cancer cells in the digestive tract

Red Pepper - digestive stimulant, anti-oxidant, supports bile functions of the liver and stimulates metabolism

Salt - an essential nutrient, regulates sodium/potassium fluid balance in the cell, is necessary for the muscles to relax and contract as well as for transmission of nerve impulses. Salt is essential to the formation of HCL, the digestive acid needed by the stomach for the breakdown of food. Industrially refined salt usually contains other chemicals and additives and has been stripped of most of its natural mineral content. Natural salts, unrefined, such as sea salt, pink salt or celtic grey salt are healthier choices. Processed foods account for three quarters of the salt in the modern American diet. The salt shaker on the table is rarely the problem. When sodium levels are restricted due to kidney disease, eliminating the processed food is more important than any other form of salt restriction.

Cilantro - aids digestion, member of carrot family, use fresh

Nutmeg - supports circulation

Thyme - anti-spasmodic, anti-cough when used as liquid drops (thyme oil) or tea

Clove - anti-oxidant, warming, pain relief for tooth pain or arthritis

Vanilla - calming, relaxing, supports nerves

Cardamom - improves digestion

Parsley - detoxes liver and blood, improves digestion and lowers blood pressure

Sage - detoxes blood, astringent, anti-cough when used as tea

Bay Leaf - improves digestion of beef or lamb

Mushrooms - shiitake - anti-cancer, anti-fungal, host defense potentiators

Oyster mushrooms - host defense potentiators

When choosing spices, always choose high quality over low price. Basil, oregano, mint and cilantro are important to use organic. To reap the benefits of these healing spices, incorporate them into your diet. Create a living relationship with them. Discover their personalities and their hidden powers.

VIBRATION FREQUENCIES IN FOOD

Everything vibrates. Rates of vibration produce color, form and density. The human organism is a symphony of vibrations - some are held in our emotions or our mental outlook; some held in our cells and organs. This energy body is giving expression to certain qualities that my intuition interprets in the language of emotions. All that we consume vibrates in certain patterns and wave lengths that constitute a language between the cells of the food and the cells of our body.

Fruits
Apples - pleasure
Apricots - amused
Blueberries - amused
Cantaloupe - self-esteem
Cherries - kindness
Dates - innocence
Figs - reverence
Grapes - pleasure
   grocery grapes with pesticide - grief
   after salt soak - inspired
Grapefruit - reverence
Honeydew - equality
Lemons - kindness
Nectarines - reverence
Oranges - intellectualization, brilliance
Pineapple - pleasure
Plums - sensitive
Pomegranate - confidence
Prunes - care
Raisins - pleasure
Raspberries - reverence

Strawberries - adoration
   grocery berries with with pesticides - intolerant
   after salt water soak reads - inspired

Spices
Anise - kindness
Basil - pleasure
Cardamon - self-esteem
Chili Pepper - kindness
Cinnamon - responsible
Curry - pleasure
Garlic - self-esteem

Vegetables
Artichoke - consideration
Beets - raw - consideration
   cooked - kindness
Bell Pepper - raw - consideration
   cooked - kindness
Bok Choy - cooked - love
Broccoli - raw - self-esteem
   cooked - equality

Asparagus - raw - intellectualization
   cooked - self esteem
Cabbage - raw - security
   cooked - confidence
Cauliflower - raw - reverence
   cooked - love
Carrots - raw - self-esteem
   cooked - equality
Celery - raw - amused
   cooked - not amused
Cilantro - pleasure
Cucumbers - intellectualization
Eggplant - undependable
Green Beans - raw - confidence
   cooked - not confident
Lettuce - romaine and iceberg - kindness
   red leaf - consideration
Mushrooms - responsible
Olives - black - equality, green - self-esteem
Onions - raw - sensitive
   cooked - responsible
Potato - baked - divine love
Sauerkraut - confidence
Sweet Potato - cooked - love
Spinach - raw - self-esteem
   cooked - interest
Tomatoes - raw - responsible
   cooked - affection

Meats
Organic Grass fed Chicken - self-esteem
Organic Grass fed Beef - pleasure
Lamb - equality
Pork - equality
Turkey - equality
Wild Caught Salmon - responsible

Spices
Ginger - kindness
Mint - kindness
Pepper - pleasure
Salt - self-esteem
Sugar - reverence
Vanilla - sensitive

Grains - Cooked
Basmati rice - responsible
Corn - self-esteem
Lentils - consideration
Oats – self-esteem
Wheat - responsible
Soy - responsible

Grains - GMO
Rice - not creative
Corn - low self-esteem
Wheat - anguish
Soy - anguish
BT Potatoes - anguish

Beverage
Cocoa - grace
Coffee - self-esteem
Black tea - self-esteem
Green tea - equality

Meats - GMO
Antibiotic and grain fed Chickens - shame
Turkey Antibiotic & GMO fed- shame
Grain fed Beef - fear
Farm raised Salmon - shame

Nuts
Almonds - self-esteem
   cooked - equality
Cashews - reverence
   cooked - pleasure

Macadamia - amused
   cooked - defensiveness
Peanuts - rude
   cooked - self-esteem x 7 days then changes
   to intolerant
Pecans - reverence
   cooked - love
Pistachios - liveliness
   cooked - amused
Walnuts - sympathy
   cooked - liveliness

Dairy

Milk, whole organic - compassion
Butter - creative
Cheeses - sympathy
Sour Cream - inspired
Homemade Yogurt - inspired

Oils

Olive - self-esteem
   cooked - desire
Canola - unkind
   cooked - unkind
Corn - equality
   cooked - divine
Cottonseed - sarcastic
   cooked - uninspired
Safflower - compassion
   cooked-intolerant
Sunflower - adoration

"If you want to find the secrets of the universe, think in terms of energy, frequency and vibration".

Nikola Tesla

WHAT IF YOU ARE VEGETARIAN OR VEGAN?

This protocol is primarily written from the perspective of an omnivore with no judgments other than the physiology of real, sustainable health. Broth is featured prominently as a protein source for raising protein levels to 30%. Changing to vegetarian broth is not an adequate substitute in the area of protein. The vegetarian broth does have benefits but there are several things which will provide more protein from non-animal sources. First and foremost, soaked raw nuts and the fresh foods made from them including dressings and nut milks. Soaking the nuts increases the amount of protein available as well as improves the quality of the protein as to ease of assimilation. A vegan could have 20% to 25% of their diet from nut based proteins. The rancid oil in roasted nuts is not good for anyone. As a primary protein source nuts should be raw. Many people are sensitive to nuts and cannot have certain ones or sometimes any at all. For them, sprouts are the best alternative protein. Most sprouts have 25 to 30% protein. Sunflower sprouts are among the highest protein sprouts and the most widely enjoyed for flavor and texture. Additionally, avocados are an excellent source of protein and healthy fats and one can benefit from eating them every day.

The outlook of the readings is to respect the vegetarian and vegan diets as spiritual practice, not a moral right or wrong and not a healthy choice. The vegetarian and vegan diets will not protect the health if they are based on primarily processed grains and convenience foods. This will lead to insulin resistance, type 2 diabetes and Alzheimer's. The spiritual practice of not consuming animal products can create health if it is based on whole fresh foods, avoids unhealthy oils, eliminates processed foods and grains and provides adequate protein. Maintaining health and the spiritual practice of vegan diet, particularly requires careful attention to balance and responsibility for meeting the body's real needs physically, as well as spiritually. There is a risk of over dependance on organic but processed convenience foods that rapidly raise blood sugar and insulin levels but do not provide lasting strength.

Our relationship with food is a social justice issue. Sustainable health is inseparable from the issues of sustainable Earth. Choosing vegan, organic, non-toxic to the planet, and choosing regional food locally sourced, these are all important factors in the hunger issues of our time. These choices influence food, fuel, health and finance. Currently, one billion people are hungry at all times. In the U.S. we throw half of our food away. We know much of it is non-nutritive fake food and we don't value it. We don't trust our food supply and we are relieved to throw it away. We have an over supply of cheap, low quality, quasi-food products in various stages of spoilage. We recognize that we are better off throwing away this unhealthy food than eating it. If we paid the real full value of wholesome, nutritious food, we would be less casual about throwing half of it away.

SUPPLEMENTS, VITAMINS, MINERALS, BOTANICALS

A significant part of my work as a medical intuitive is to provide guidance for optimal use of available supplements. The goal is a state of physical strength, health and wellness that does not require a lot of supplements, pills, powders and herbal concoctions. Many of my clients were (at the time of their first reading or consultation) taking too many supplements in a conscientious effort to make use of widely available information about each little thing, new and old, that might improve their odds of achieving better health.

The excess of supplements all together were undermining their ability to achieve the health goals intended because many of their supplements were using up hydration, lowering pH, placing extra burden on the body's processing systems including digestive, kidneys and liver and providing no essential benefits. There are many marketing miracles being widely sold today which do not provide the claimed health benefits.

There are also some real miracles available to those who need them. The answers that I receive during attunements for my clients often do not agree with widely held and widely marketed views of our time. The guidance I receive and then put forward is often contrary to where logic and reason would seem to lead and yet, working backwards from the intuitive answers I receive, it is often possible to discover new logic and new aspects of reason that explain and support the use of the intuitively guided answers.

The most commonly needed supplements are probiotics to support digestive health. Infants, children, teenagers, adults and the elderly all benefit from wise use of well indicated probiotics. Probiotics can improve digestion and reduce colic in newborns. They can reduce allergies and ear infections in children and they help the body eliminate candida overgrowth and food born toxins including arsenic and glyphosate. The body makes its own probiotics from fermented foods like olives, pickles, sauerkraut and kimchi.

Vitamin C, Vitamin B complex, and CoQ10 are among the most frequently indicated recommendations throughout the approximately 9,000 intuitive readings. CoQ10 does not come up as a positive recommendation in children's readings or even young adults, but from about age

50 and up it seems almost universally indicated to protect the brain and heart, as well as, increase vitality and oxygenation. Oregano oil is frequently recommended to clear infections including from the lungs, upper respiratory, sinus, teeth and even nail fungus.

Colloidal silver never gets a positive recommendation in the readings for fighting infections because it reads as a toxin in the human body. It opens up pathways in the body which allow the infection to penetrate to deeper organs and systems and be suppressed there. It relieves symptoms at more superficial levels while creating more serious problems in the constitutional health.

Iron, Magnesium, Calcium, Zinc and Copper are frequently (sometimes Iodine) indicated as beneficial in the readings, but rarely are all of them indicated for the same individual. Specific forms of each of these have been recommended, most frequently because of accessibility through the body's weakened assimilative processes.

Magnesium, for instance, assimilates well through the skin in Epsom salts baths and assimilates well as a topical liquid or spray. However, in the latter form it is known to sting and burn, particularly if there are skin sores or rash, where as the Epsom salts bath is more calming and soothing. For internal use, magnesium also is available in different forms that do not assimilate equally well. The magnesium powder called Natural Calm which is mixed in hot water, assimilates quickly and efficiently (in just minutes) while magnesium tablets assimilate more slowly and less efficiently. This is important because available magnesium lowers anxiety, improves brain function, calms nerves and builds strong bones. A high stress lifestyle, smoking, alcohol, prescription medications and an acid forming diet can use up enormous amounts of magnesium very quickly.

The National Institute of Health has identified 13 vitamins and 14 mineral elements as essential for human health. Current estimates suggest that over 90% of Americans are deficient in one or more of these essential nutrients because both humans and their livestock no longer eat natural diets. Better quality food, fresh organic fruits and vegetables, high quality proteins and healthy oils are all more important than any attempt to compensate for not eating wisely.

You cannot consistently eat a poor quality diet and successfully make up for it with supplements. Even the best supplements, wisely chosen and consistently used, will not overcome the challenges and toll taken on the body due to lifestyle factors of chronic high stress, insufficient exercise and inadequate relaxation and deep restful sleep. Each of these factors can be partially addressed by targeting specific nutrients for extra support but, in the absence of relaxed states of comfort and happiness and consistent consumption of fresh natural wholesome foods, the health of the body will weaken and deteriorate in predictable patterns. Therapeutic doses of specific nutrients are higher than amounts designated as maintenance doses for meeting minimum daily requirements and therapeutic doses are safely used to support returning the body's stores of these nutrients and effective functional access to these nutrients to optimum levels.

Choosing supplements wisely is becoming increasingly difficult as the industry brings new products to market, changes the name on products, discontinues products you've relied on, and changes the story of who needs what, how much and why. In general, liquid forms of supplements tend to assimilate more readily. Floradix liquid vitamin and mineral supplements and magnesium powder mixed with warm water like Natural Calm are excellent examples of supplements used in liquid form that are the best products available for their intended purposes. Second after liquid versions, capsule forms of supplements are more readily assimilated than tablet forms. The more tablets one takes, the more likely that some of them sit in the gut too long and do little to promote improved health. Third, it matters very much what brand you use, and cheaper is almost never better. Good products, the best products, are frequently available at a discount off of full retail and that is the best way to buy them; but, the cheapest brands and versions of vitamins, minerals and herbal supplements which are widely available in drug stores and grocery stores will not be as good a product and will not produce the best results.

Synthetic versions of supplements are never as good as natural forms. Vitamin E for instance is now widely marketed as a mixed tocopherol because it is much less expensive to produce and it is presumed the body can convert the mixed tocopherol to the one the body needs which is pure d-alpha tocopherol. It is more effective just to supplement with the one the body can use without any conversion, because if the body's fat metabolism is compromised or liver function is weak, the body may have trouble getting enough fat soluble nutrients, including vitamin E.

Food based supplements made from whole fruit and vegetable concentrates are more bioavailable than supplements that are not made from whole food. Food based supplements also contain probiotics and other naturally occurring co-factors such as enzymes and bioflavonoids which further enhance their effectiveness. Protein powder is one seemingly food based supplement that never reads positive in any of my many attunements to it. Even the very best brand, all natural, organic, plant based or whey based protein powders read negative for everybody. They are a highly refined, highly processed food product that is designed to be stored for many months before it is finally used. The product you buy off the shelf today may already be 8 to 10 months old from the date of manufacture. I have checked over five hundred times for different clients and on maybe a dozen different products and in all cases the protein powders read that they metabolized at about 27% to 29% sugar and only 20% to 22% protein. That's not a protein supplement, it's a marketing miracle - a product that sells spectacularly well even though it doesn't do what you are using it for.

There are two excellent ways to supplement protein with whole natural foods that will increase strength and speed recovery because they do not compromise healthy hydration and pH. For non-vegetarians the best choice is high protein broth, homemade not processed. For vegetarians the best protein supplement is raw nut cream made from soaked raw almonds or cashews. It can be added to one's raw juice to make a high protein smoothie or eaten as a dip, a dressing or a pie filling.

The references and information in this chapter will not cover many essential nutrients that are rarely recommended in the reading for supplementation. In many cases, that may be because that element is not the one causing physiological mayhem, but in some cases it may be that supplements of that element rarely provide the solution to the causal problem. For instance, my list will cover magnesium because it is one of the most frequently needed supplements of our time. My list will not explain molybdenum, manganese or even individual B vitamins because these do not appear in the readings as recommended in that form. Vitamin B is consistently recommended in the form of vitamin B complex containing all 11 B vitamins.

Among those 11 B vitamins only Folic Acid is frequently recommended for supplementation as a single nutrient. For those who need the benefits of multiple supplements, dividing the doses into two or three different times of day works better in the body than taking many capsules all at one time each day. There are many good brands of supplements available. I usually find that even good brands are not always equally good in all their products, so I use and recommend many different brands including Bluebonnet, Flora, Rainbow Light, Solgar, Thompsons, New Chapter, Source Naturals, Jarrow and doTerra.

Natural Hormone Supplements

At about age 44, most of my clients read positive for needing support with hormone balance. I notice a change in people at about that year of life. A moment comes when assessment of the realities of life in one's personal experience begs some kind of conclusion about going on or not going on and how to integrate with what life and death require of us. Often there is a state of physical burnout around this time of life. Years and years of burning the candle at both ends in pursuit of your hopes and dreams in areas of personal accomplishment, career development and parenting leave most of us depleted energetically, both physically and psychologically. This is a time of reassessing priorities and the outcome of that assessment has very significant consequences not only in the realm of how we will live but in how and when we will die.

This period of self assessment seems to be specifically triggered by falling levels of sex hormones. The adrenals make 50% of the hormones for the body. The adrenals become exhausted and inefficient at maintaining optimal hormone levels. Both cortisol and progesterone use the same hormone precursor. When elevated stress levels persist long term, more of the precursor is used up making cortisol and less is available for making progesterone. For females, before about age 44, that stress response from the body was mitigated by the body's alternate source of progesterone, the corpus luteum and the processes of ovulation. A woman who is not ovulating does not have that additional significant source of progesterone. Historically, there has until recently been an additional source of progesterone through a natural diet because all raw fruits and vegetables contain it, but we don't eat very much raw food anymore. The modern American diet reads about 5% raw food. To optimize hormone balance through diet would require about 50% raw food.

Progesterone is a safe hormone that is needed in abundance. It is necessary for healthy bones, skin, sleep and circulation as well as reproduction. When all progesterone receptors are filled, the body will use it to make other essential hormones including estrogen. For that reason, a woman taking Tomoxafin is not a candidate for using an over the counter hormone cream of any kind. Those who are on prescription medications to prevent the body from making estrogen as a preventative approach to cancer can only use hormone supplements that are prescribed by their doctor. Because I am a consultant for natural health care, most of my clients will not have chosen this medical approach to preventing cancer. I find in the readings that most women over age 44 will have the same percent of excess cortisol as they have of deficient progesterone. Commonly, if the cortisol reads near 25% high the progesterone level will read near 25% low.

Increasing available progesterone quickly through topical application can provide much needed support for vein wall health and circulation, support for bone health in manifestations of arthritis and osteoporosis, heal extreme dry skin and promote deeper, longer sleep. Progesterone is a fat soluble hormone that is absorbed readily through the skin and less efficiently as an oral supplement. It can be used locally at the site of application for targeted relief as well as benefiting the entire body systemically from brains to bones and everything in between.

Hormone replacement therapy does not supplement progesterone alone. Hormone replacement therapy, when necessary, should always be guided by a medical professional using bio-identical hormones. Bio-identical means that they are not extracted from horse urine. This kind of hormone replacement is discouraged even by the medical profession for women over age 65 because it is associated with increased cancer rates. Hormone replacement therapy is best limited to four years duration or less and the time used to make necessary changes to support better health.

Men also show a lowering level of hormones at about the same age as women. This is due to diet (about 50%) and also due to environmental chemical exposures. Men can protect hormone health by not eating the industrialized meats and dairy that are loaded with hormone residue from the methods used to produce them. Also avoiding the chemical burden in personal care products, cleaning products, pesticides, herbicides and the crops they were used on (GMO) is becoming increasingly necessary because exposure is cumulative and exponentially increasing.

Environmental toxins in the soil, water, air and oceans appear to be weakening the healthy development of male hormones in fish, frogs and other vulnerable species, including humans, thus rendering them incapable of reproduction and perhaps, especially in the case of mankind, incapable of sex or being influenced in sexual orientation and gender identity by the chemical overload. The increase in same sex and bi-sexual attraction is more of a chemical phenomena than it is a social awakening. The awakening is that our relationship with the elements of the planet have evolved us to this current state and there is no individual or group who can be faulted for it. This is the state of what is and it requires of us to be dealt with for what it is without blame or criticism. The 'times they are a changing' and we, as a global population, are as responsible for this as we are for global warming.

BPA, or bi-phenylalanine, is an estrogen mimicking polymer which has been used for many years to make plastic, (think plastic bottles). Estrogen mimicking means that the cells of the body respond to this polymer as if it were the hormone estrogen. That effect on the cells of the body is why BPA is considered to cause or promote cancer. Unnaturally high estrogen levels stimulate growth in cancer cells. Current research indicates the presence of BPA toxins in 92% of Americans. It is also widely found in breast milk. Plastic is now by law required to be labeled as to BPA content, but the planet and our lives are inundated by plastics made before this danger was recognized.

Hormones profoundly affect our experience as human beings from sense of well being to sense of identity. Thyroid hormones which regulate metabolism and energy production from the breakdown of fats profoundly affect the normal process of breaking down and eliminating unhealthy cells. Regulation of this process of cell death, called apoptosis, is an essential defense against cancer. Iodine deficiency is present with about 70% of all cancers. Iodine chemistry also plays a significant role in prostate health and about 50% of men with enlarged prostates need supplemental iodine. Bromine, which is mostly found in processed foods such as bromated flours, blocks the absorption of iodine in the body. Iodine assimilation is also inhibited by consumption of raw kale, raw cabbage, brussels sprouts and cauliflower.

When Are Supplements Beneficial?

Several specific sets of circumstances usually warrant judicious use of supplements. Increasing age is associated with weakening of digestion and assimilation as well as generalized decline of organs and systems due to the wear and tear of life's demands. Supplementation is often a fast efficient way to provide additional support for increasing energy, vitality and cognitive functions. Any diagnosis of acute or chronic illness also lends itself to specific nutrients and botanical supplements to aid in restoring health and wellness. Any trauma, accident, surgery or broken bones is also intensely demanding nutritionally to provide the cells with the materials necessary to rebuild healthy tissues.

Similarly, pregnancy and nursing (lactation) are nutritionally demanding at a level that is difficult to meet adequately through diet alone. The health of both mother and baby are significantly improved by taking specific well indicated supplements. Additionally, states of chronic high stress, anxiety, grief or loss cause a higher level of demand for certain nutrients particularly to protect the brain, nervous system, immune system and adrenals.

Many could reasonably go through long periods of health and well being when they take no supplements at all, however a change of circumstance may well call for additional support to meet the challenge and optimize the body's healing response. Smoking, drinking, over the counter drugs and prescription medications also increase nutritional demands beyond what can be compensated for by diet alone. Even regular vigorous exercise, which is a healthy activity, increases the nutritional needs of the body to replace minerals lost through exertion and the nutritive components to rebuild healthy cells, tissues and organs and replenish vital stores of energy.

Taking supplements that are not well matched to your needs or that are not highly effective not only costs more money, it also uses up much needed hydration and lowers pH when 3 or more daily supplements fail to deliver the intended benefit for which they were chosen. Health and wellness depend on far more than just getting all the right supplements. Taking even the very best and most needed supplements is only a partial solution when it comes to maintaining or regaining health, and it is not enough unless it is part of a healthy lifestyle that creates balance and happiness.

Top 8 Supplements - in order of frequency with which they are recommended.

1. Probiotics
2. Vitamin C
3. CoQ10
4. Omegas
5. Vitamin B Complex
6. Magnesium
7. Vitamin E
8. Vitamin A

Top 8 Mistakes - using supplements for extra support

1. Gluten free processed foods - are not health foods and promote insulin resistance, always make homemade
2. Not consuming enough water with supplements, promotes dehydration
3. Protein powder - more sugar than protein, promotes acidosis
4. Taking too many supplements - 4 supplements is better than 10
5. Poor quality probiotics - use the best, use refrigerated
6. Not addressing the underlying reasons making supplements necessary

7. Not eliminating supplements during periods when they are no longer needed. The consequence may be failure to create those periods of going off of supplements
8. Taking tablets instead of capsules or liquids. Using forms that pass through the body without assimilating. Always choose bioavailability.

Vitamin A

Vitamin A is made in the liver from beta carotene. Liver weakness, thyroid weakness and diabetes all inhibit absorption of beta carotene and conversion to vitamin A. Antibiotics, laxatives, steroids, cholesterol lowering medication and birth control pills all interfere with assimilation of vitamin A. This vitamin has important antioxidant properties that protect cells from disease including cancer and is vital to repair of body tissues and wound healing. Vitamin A is also needed for vision health, especially for good night vision and prevention of cataracts. Inability to digest fats and medications that block the production of stomach acid contribute to vitamin A deficiency because stomach acids are a catalyst for converting beta carotene to its useable form called vitamin A. Lycopene and lutein are in the beta carotene family. Food sources of this vitamin include carrots, cantaloupe, sweet potatoes, winter squash, pumpkin, papaya, peaches, apricots, watercress, asparagus, beets and spinach. Fish liver oils and animal liver in general is a rich source of vitamin A. This is a fat soluble nutrient that is stored in the liver and can accumulate at toxic levels when supplemented at over 10,000 International Units daily. The recommended amount is usually 5,000 I.U.'s.

Vitamin B Complex

Most discussions of vitamin B Complex functions in the body are broken down so as to highlight the action of each of its component elements, but the B vitamins work together and a deficiency is often best relieved by providing all the elements of B vitamins in specific proportions of these elements to each other called B Complex. The B vitamins are widely recognized for their role in relieving stress and depression. In fact, the label often says stress formula on the bottle, indicating that the FDA has approved its marketing for this use. Most of the B vitamins have functions relating to metabolizing food to produce energy. B vitamins also regulate circulatory health, blood vessel dilation and blood oxygen levels. B vitamins regulate cell division and have essential functions allowing the body to use iron and produce red blood cells and improve oxygenation. The brain and spinal cord use large amounts of B vitamins which improve memory and protect healthy vision. Alcohol, cigarettes and oral contraceptives produce vitamin B deficiency. B vitamins are found in many foods including fruits, vegetables, milk, meat and eggs. Lecithin, also called phosphatidyl choline (PC), protects nerves and brain cells and is in the B vitamin family. PABA (used to protect the skin from sun over exposure) is a constituent of folic acid. Folic acid is a micro nutrient and yet its effects are among the most far reaching for brain and nervous system health.

Vitamin C

Vitamin C was the first of the vitamins to be extensively researched. Current research indicates that probably half the population of America is consuming too little vitamin C to meet the body's minimum needs. Vitamin C is recommended frequently in the intuitive readings in large amounts. It is recommended both orally and intravenously. Vitamin C supports immune functions and is particularly recommended for recovery from pneumonia, colds, flu and upper respiratory infections. Vitamin C is essential to the process by which cells burn energy. Vitamin C helps lower blood pressure and improves circulation, thereby reducing risk of heart attack and stroke. Vitamin C helps protect the eyes from glaucoma, cataracts and macular degeneration.

Smoking depletes the body of vitamin C, which is one of the ways smoking promotes wrinkles and respiratory weakness. The body cannot make vitamin C. It is a water soluble vitamin and stays in the body only a couple of hours before any excess is excreted in the urine. The fact that you excrete excess vitamin C in the urine has been used to draw the conclusion that large doses are thus wasted. However, this process of peeing out excess vitamin C allows it to concentrate where it is needed most - in the adrenals and kidneys. The adrenals are the primary user and storehouse of vitamin C in the body. Adrenal exhaustion and adrenal insufficiency often respond with rapid improvement following intravenous vitamin C infusions. Pneumonia and cancer, both of which produce adrenal exhaustion, are also significantly relieved by I.V. vitamin C.

Vitamin C is also necessary for the absorption of the essential nutrients iron and copper which are necessary for healthy blood and circulation. Vitamin C is also significant for oral and dental health as a support for healthy gums, teeth and bones. Sources of vitamin C include all citrus fruits, strawberries, papaya, spinach, green peppers and chili peppers. Quercetin and pycnogenols are also in the vitamin C family and have significant applications for support of immune health.

Quercetin is also called a bioflavonoid, a form of antioxidant. It has anti-hyper immune properties, anti-histamine and anti-inflammatory functions. Quercetin significantly reduces hyper immune response and allergic reactions including watery itchy eyes, nasal congestion, sneezing, welts, rashes and hives. It is needed in large amount to produce this relief of allergic symptoms and it is very short acting. Amounts of 3 to 4 grams every 2 hours for a day or two is usually enough to relieve an acute episode of allergies. For the hyper immune response of leaky gut syndrome a longer period of supplements is required. Two to four grams per dose three times a day for 3 to 6 months may be required for symptom control. Quercetin also lowers blood pressure and relieves prostate inflammation. Quercertin is found in onions, apples, cherries, red grapes, broccoli, garlic and even black tea.

Pycnogenols are antioxidants with powerful anti-inflammatory and pain relief functions that may provide relief for some forms of arthritis, but it is not often recommended in the intuitive readings.

Vitamin D

Also called vitamin D3, vitamin D deficiency has become prevalent in the last 15 years. Scientists have recently concluded that as many as 3 out of 4 Americans may be deficient in vitamin D. There are two reasons for this widespread shortage but one of them is not getting discussed enough. Vitamin D is synthesized in the body in response to absorption of direct sunlight. Just 15 minutes per day of sun exposure allows the liver and kidneys to convert the needed vitamin D to its active form which increases calcium absorption in the body. However, because vitamin D is essential for calcium transport it is called upon not only for the healthy mineralization of teeth and bones, it is also necessary to the process of withdrawing minerals from the bones to buffer acidosis.

When pH is chronically in the acidic range the body is further challenged by the mixed message to both lay down minerals in the bones to provide needed strength and pull minerals from the bones to buffer the pH. This state of disruption can use as much as 400% more than the amount of vitamin D needed to transport minerals when the pH is maintained within normal range. Diseases which normally manifest with significant acidosis and therefore exhibit vitamin D deficiencies include cancer, diabetes and fibromyalgia. Supplementing with vitamin D does not do enough to heal the disease. Only return to normal pH will do that. The recommended amount of oral supplement of vitamin D is usually 1,000 I.U.'s to 2,000 I.U.'s daily. Those with significant kidney or liver weakness may have poor utilization of vitamin D. Diuretics, cholesterol lowering drugs, antacid and steroids (including prednisone) also interfere with utilization of vitamin D.

Vitamin E

This is a fat soluble vitamin which has anti-aging effects due to improved circulation and its function in wound healing and skin repair. Vitamin E prevents cell damage and regulates normal blood clotting. Vitamin E supports healthy blood flow to the heart and protects against atherosclerosis, the build up of obstructions in the blood vessels attributed to "bad" cholesterol. Vitamin E supports male fertility as well as healthy pregnancy and birth. It's important in muscle and nerve maintenance and the formation of red blood cells. Vitamin E is present in cold pressed healthy oils, raw seeds and all raw nuts and dark green leafy vegetables. The usual dose is 400 I.U.'s two times a day. Pure d-alpha tocopherol works better than mixed tocopherols.

CoQ10

Coenzyme Q10 is essential to the production of the basic energy of every cell. The body makes CoQ10, but only if you exercise. CoQ10 is especially important for healthy heart functions and optimal brain circulation. It supports improved oxygenation, increased energy and enhances mental clarity. CoQ10 levels diminish with age and are also reduced by cholesterol lowering drugs. CoQ10 is an excellent support for recovery from jet lag. Treatment of severe challenges such as cancer, heart disease and Alzheimer's requires large doses in the range of 300 to 400 mgs twice daily. CoQ10 protects against cortisol binding in the brain.

Complete Omega's

Supplementing with essential fatty acids from fish oil, flax oil and walnuts is one of the best ways to support both brain health and heart health. These fatty acids, also called omega's are found in the highest amounts in healthy brains where they support transmission of nerve impulses. They reduce inflammation, help keep blood pressure in normal range and improve memory. They also benefit arthritis which is an inflammatory disease. These essential fatty acids are needed in the formation of the fatty acid cell membrane covering every cell in the body. Unhealthy fats do not provide the essential fatty acids necessary to feed the brain and the heart and make healthy cells. We do not have enough healthy oils in our diet, and after age 45 when we enter a phase of needing to rebuild and recover from life up to that point, this is one of the most frequently needed supplements of our time. Omega's are significant for relief of depression, anxiety and obsessive compulsive tendencies.

The usual dose is 2 to 4 grams daily taken as a divided dose of 1 to 2 grams morning and evening.

Magnesium

Magnesium is the mineral element most frequently recommended in the intuitive health readings. Leading symptoms of magnesium deficiency are anxiety and loss of ability to cope with normal stress. Magnesium is critical to the health of bones, muscles and nerves. Because of the acid forming diet that is our cultural norm, our bodies use additional magnesium to raise pH. Secondly, because of chronic unrelenting stress our bodies use extra magnesium to relax muscles and lower the stress response. Magnesium relieves leg cramps and promotes healthy sleep cycles.

Magnesium is stored in the bones for later use as needed by muscles and nerves. This storehouse of magnesium becomes depleted and colon health is jeopardized because bowels become sluggish. Constipation is a leading indicator for magnesium deficiency. Magnesium helps the body absorb calcium and it helps regulate blood sugar.

Natural Calm by Natural Vitality is the best selling magnesium supplement in the world. This powdered form of magnesium, when dissolved in warm water, assimilates better than any other form available. The best food sources of magnesium are raw nuts and green vegetables, fruits, meats, salmon and seeds. Smoking, alcohol, medications, processed foods and even strenuous exercise all contribute to magnesium deficiency.

Calcium

Calcium is the most abundant mineral in the body. Calcium is called a macro-nutrient because the body needs so much of it. In fact, we need three times as much calcium as magnesium. Magnesium is essential in calcium transport so lack of magnesium renders calcium unavailable to the nerve cells, the brain and bones. Calcium makes muscles contract and is an excitatory element in neurochemistry. Magnesium makes muscles relax and is a calming element in the nervous system and brain chemistry. Both of these minerals circulate in the blood and are essential to bone mineralization, to the activation of nerve impulses to send messages across nerve synapses, and can be stored in the bones and then later be extracted from bones and muscle cells to return to the blood stream to buffer acidosis.

The emotional frequency of calcium is confidence and calcium deficiency produces anxiety and depression. The frequency of magnesium is security. When these two minerals are available in adequate amounts they calm the nerves, relieve anxiety and promote better sleep. Calcium also has functions relative to blood clotting and blood pressure. Calcium absorption takes place in both the small and large intestine and can be more bioavailable in the presence of probiotics. These two together make the pH in the intestines more alkaline. Processed foods, carbonated beverages, alcohol and caffeine all cause loss of calcium through the urine.

Calcium is widely available in healthy foods including almonds, dairy, fish and leafy greens as well as meat, poultry and eggs. The recommended dose ranges from 1 to 2 grams daily taken as a divided dose, half in the morning and half in the evening. Raw calcium, coral calcium and calcium citrate are recommended forms.

The amino acid lysine is needed for calcium absorption. This is significant for anyone with herpes who will likely need lysine supplementation at least during acute herpes out breaks. The hormones estrogen and progesterone promote strong mineralization of bones.

Iron

Iron is a micro-nutrient that makes up the largest amount of mineral element in the blood. It is frequently needed by growing children and women of childbearing age. It is almost universally beneficial as a supplement during the last 8 weeks of pregnancy when the fetal liver is storing iron. Iron deficiency occurs in part with any degree of malnutrition because the body requires vitamins A, B, C and copper to absorb iron. Excessive bleeding causes iron deficiency, but so does a normal growth spurt which uses up large amounts of this mineral for energy production and for the manufacture of red blood cells.

Iron deficiency impairs cognitive development and contributes to irritability and depression due to reduced oxygen carrying capacity of the blood. The brain is especially affected. Iron is more bioavailable from food based sources and less likely to promote constipation in that form. Iron is found in leafy greens, almonds, beets, dried prunes and raisins, dates and other fruits as well as fish, meat, and poultry. Floradix liquid iron with herbs (available gluten-free) is the form of iron most frequently recommended in the readings. Gaia Plant Force Iron is also excellent.

Iron supplementation is almost never indicated for grown men because they store iron more effectively than women and children. Iron levels must be within a certain range and excess iron is also undesirable and can result in cell damage increasing risk of cancer and heart disease. Those whose iron levels are too high benefit from vitamin E to safely regulate their iron levels.

Iodine

Iodine is a micronutrient, needed in only trace amounts. Though the dose is measured in millionths of a gram, this element is crucial to maintaining thyroid health and regulation of metabolism, especially fat metabolism. Iodine chemistry plays a role in energy production, temperature regulation and hormone balance. Interest in iodine supplementation increases whenever there is massive leakage of radio-active elements or nuclear disaster. It is true that iodine supplementation is significant in protecting the thyroid because when the iodine receptors are already filled, the thyroid will not take up radioactive iodine. However, nuclear disasters leak many other radioactive elements that iodine supplementation does not provide protection from. Swelling of the thyroid gland, at the base of the throat, is called goiter. It is an indication both to supplement with iodine and to have your thyroid checked by your doctor if the swelling persists for 2 weeks. Raw kale, raw cabbage, raw cauliflower and brussels sprouts all inhibit the absorption of iodine. Iodine is found in all ocean plants and sea life. The filtered, odorless, tasteless drops may be your safest source.

Zinc

Zinc is an essential trace mineral in every cell of the body. Zinc helps regulate insulin levels and is important in the treatment of diabetes. Zinc is essential to immune functions and has a role in over 300 enzyme actions. Zinc supports wound healing including cold sores and acne. It is also significant for vision and prevention of macular degeneration. Zinc is necessary for production of testosterone and prostate health. Zinc regulates levels of vitamin E in the blood and is required for protein synthesis. Zinc supplementation is a moderate dose of 15 mgs to 30 mgs. because levels above optimum interfere with copper absorption and immune functions. Zinc and copper act together to form superoxy dismutase, a powerful anti-oxidant. Zinc deficiency causes eczema, acne, hair loss, absence of menses, infertility and loss of taste and smell. Food sources of zinc include oysters, seafood, pecans, raw sunflower seeds and raw pumpkin seeds. Zinc helps the liver eliminate toxic metals including lead. To improve insulin resistance, combine with alpha lipoic acid. After age 50 the body absorbs less zinc. 30 mgs daily may be necessary to support prostate health for men in this age range.

Copper

Copper is a micronutrient that is essential to healthy heart functions, arteries, blood vessels and red blood cells. Copper increases absorption of iron. Copper is needed for fat metabolism and normal insulin functions. Copper is also essential to bone health and the formation of collagen and bone matrix. Copper deficiency promotes osteoporosis.

Copper is needed in specific proportion to the levels of both vitamin C and zinc. High doses of oral vitamin C (about 20 grams a day for a week) will reduce copper and zinc availability. Copper deficiency contributes to aneurism, anemia and bleeding irregularities including heart attack. There is no RDA for copper. The usual dose is quite small, usually 3 mgs. Food sources of copper include raw almonds, raw walnuts, dried fruit, raw honey, mushrooms and kelp. High blood sugar reduces availability of copper and thereby contributes to anemia.

Probiotics

The intestinal track is the body's first line of defense against disease. About one third of Americans, 95 million people, experience digestive difficulties. Without proper digestion, nutrients can't be absorbed and toxins accumulate. Probiotics are beneficial bacteria that live in the gut. They fight dangerous bacteria including food poisoning, inhibit yeast overgrowth in the intestines, chelate out environmental toxins like arsenic and glyphosate and support normal bowel movements. The probiotic reuteri helps assimilation of vitamin D.

The body doesn't make its own probiotics unless provided with the necessary elements including raw food fiber from fruits and vegetables as prebiotics and fermented foods that have not been pasteurized. Pasteurization kills probiotics which are temperature sensitive. Many must be kept refrigerated. Homemade pickles and sauerkraut are excellent sources of healthy probiotics. The functions of the upper digestive tract are very different from the functions of the lower digestive tract or colon and they require different strains of probiotics to complete those functions. For this reason, high quality probiotics often have several different strains in each formula. Most people need to supplement with probiotics. Men, women, children and infants all need this extra support because of environmental toxins, food toxins and weak digestive health due to diet, stress and genetics. They can be taken with or without food several times throughout the day.

Antibiotics kill probiotics and restoring normal gut flora after any course of antibiotics is essential. Lack of sufficient probiotics can cause colic, abdominal gas, bloating and constipation. Acidophilus is also needed after diarrhea. Lactobacillus acidophilus inhibits the bacteria (H. pylori) that cause ulcers.

Lactobacillus and bifido bacteria protect against intestinal parasites. Oral contraceptives can disrupt the balance of healthy gut flora contributing to yeast overgrowth called candida. The probiotic reuteri is specific for fighting yeast. Probiotics are used to treat diverticulitis and they help make vitamin K in the intestines which is necessary for bone health. Probiotics help with the breakdown and digestion of milk proteins and are beneficial to anyone on a milk based diet, which is usually all infants and children and some adults, especially the elderly.

Enzymes

Enzymes are proteins, the building blocks of life. There are thousands of enzymes maintaining body functions. They are necessary for digestion of food, tissue repair and elimination of toxins. The body makes enzymes and gets enzymes from raw food. Most reactions in the cells are triggered by these essential proteins. Cooked food does not contain these enzymes. The more raw food you eat, the less likely you are to need supplemental enzymes.

The best known enzymes are the digestive enzymes. Because the pancreas weakens on the high blood glucose diet, the digestive enzymes produced by the pancreas diminish and the body is less able to break down food, especially carbohydrates. Usually when an enzyme supplement is chosen, it is for digestive weakness. Digestive enzymes help relieve abdominal bloating, stomach discomfort due to the pressure of gas and constipation. Digestive enzymes specifically contain lipase to break down fats, protease to break down proteins, amylase to break down carbohydrates and lactose to break down milk. All of these enzymes are available from plant source called aspergillus. We are not able to synthetically produce enzymes.

The enzymes supplement used most after the digestive complex would be SOD or superoxy dismutase. SOD is a superlative antioxidant which revitalizes cells and has anti-aging functions at the cellular level. Enzymes are anti-inflammatory agents which may be well indicated for most degenerative diseases including cancer and arthritis. These enzymes are especially concentrated in wheat grass and barley green.

SUPPLEMENTS

GABA - a neuro-nutrient that promotes relaxation and reduces anxiety. Its action in the brain is calming and promotes clarity (1,000 mgs daily)

L-tryptophan - an essential amino acid that supports relaxation and sleep, it is active in the synthesis of melatonin and serotonin. It supports nervous system health, immune health and metabolism. (500 mgs daily)

5 - HTP - also an amino acid, it raises serotonin levels relieving anxiety and depression and improves sleep (100 mgs 2 x day)

Melatonin - a hormone secreted by the pineal gland which supports sleep, improving both quality and duration, and regulates the body's cycles of sleep and alertness. Caffeine, alcohol and prescription medications reduce the level and effectiveness in the body. A micro dose of 3 mg to 5 mg is sufficient.

Lithium Orotate - a neuro-nutrient, calming and balancing for the brain. Plant sourced to ensure safety. Inhibits development of both manic and depressive phases of bi-polar disorder.

Alpha lipoic acid - supports metabolism of fats, clears unhealthy fat deposits from arteries and improves heart and liver functions. Raises glutathione levels. Improves insulin resistance and mental clarity. (600 mgs 2 x day)

Oregano Oil - immune support, antimicrobial, anti-viral, anti-fungal, use for tooth infection, respiratory infection, appendicitis and toe nail fungus (3 x day, 1 to 2 caps per dose with meals) compare to GSE

MSM - plant sourced sulphur, this mineral nourishes hair, skin and nails. It is used both internally (500 to 1,000 mgs daily) and externally for skin rash, eczema and wound healing.

Flax Oil - vegetarian sourced Omega 3 fatty acids. Significant for brain support. May relieve ADHD. Use capsules or liquid.

Chinese Mushrooms - have been used for thousand of years for their healing properties. They are rich in anti-oxidants and phytonutrients. GAIA herbs is a reliable brand for high quality Chinese mushrooms in capsule form.

Shiitake - increases the number of killer cells in the lymphatic system to fight infection, support for cancer and diabetic infections. Use capsules 2 x a day, 1 to 2 grams per dose, or use fresh.

Maitake - improves glucose tolerance, inhibits growth of cancer cells and supports heart health and circulation. Use capsules rather than drops or tablet form. Use 2 grams 3 x a day - or use fresh.

Reishi - used as a tonic for vitality and longevity, supports hormone balance, emotional resilience and reduces fatigue. Use capsules instead of drops or table form, 2 grams 2 x a day.

Cordyceps - an adaptogen that provides adrenal support and strengthens endurance, builds stamina. Use capsules, 2 grams 2 x a day.

Colostrum - the precursor to mother's milk, this nutrient stimulates immune response and builds stronger defenses.

Elderberry - also called Sambucus, historically used for respiratory infection, to reduce congestion and allergies, strengthens immune response and increases fighter cells. Used as a tonic, mix elderberry syrup in a small amount of water 2 to 3 x a day.

Essiac - a combination of herbs that support immune functions and detoxing the liver, fights infection and inhibits cancer growth. Use the powder or capsule form instead of the liquid extract.

Flor-Essence - is the top selling natural detox formula. Easy to use, colorless, tasteless. Aids in the removal of toxins slowly and safely by supporting the kidneys. Improves immune function.

Lysine - the immune system uses up lots of this amino acid when fighting the herpes virus. During acute outbreaks use 1 gram 4 x a day for up to 8 days.

Hawthorne berry - vasodilator, supports circulatory and heart health, reduces angina and improves blood pressure and regulates the heartbeat. Also used to improve brain circulation and memory.

Black Walnut Tincture - all intestinal parasites, pin worms, round worm, tape worm. Used in combination with other botanicals including artemesia.

Dr. Miller's Holy Tea - combination of 5 herbs for digestive health. Relieves constipation, sluggish bowel, indigestion, bloating and acid reflux. Reduce the amount or skip a day if stool becomes too loose. Contains persimmon, malva and marshmallow leaves.

Selenium - helps prevent the formation of free radicals, stimulates the immune system. Significant for heart health and all forms of cancer. Dose is in micrograms as too much is toxic. 100 mcg's per dose 2 x a day. Best natural source is oyster mushrooms.

Maca - a Peruvian root vegetable about the size of a radish, it is related to broccoli and turnips. A true super food for depleted adrenals and thyroid, maca builds stamina and vitality and supports sexual and reproductive health for both men and woman. Raw maca powder improves hormone balance and is rich in essential fatty acids, vitamins, and minerals.

> **"All strength, all healing of every nature is the changing of vibrations from within."**
>
> **Edgar Cayce**

FREQUENCIES OF SUPPLEMENTS

Vitamin A - Tolerance

Vitamin B - Interest

Vitamin C - Kindness

Vitamin D - Confidence

Vitamin E - Responsible

CoQ10 - Attraction

Omegas - Fair

Magnesium - Safety

Calcium - Security

Iron - Self-realization

Iodine - Compassion

Probiotics - Confidence

Enzymes - Digestive tolerance

SOD - Involvement

Elderberry - Purity

Colostrum - Love

Flor-Essence - Clarity

Essiac - Self-realization

Black Walnut - Interest

Selenium - Confidence

GSE - Adoration

Colloidal silver - Defeat

Oregano oil - Not melancholy

Progesterone - Liveliness

Testosterone - Interest

Estrogen - Tolerance

GABA - Arbitrator

5HTP - Intention

L- tryptophan - Sympathy

Melatonin - Intuition

Lithium orotate - Self esteem

Alpha lipoic acid - Preserver

Reishi - Intuition

Shiitake - Intuition

Maitake - Manifestation

Cordyceps - Uphold

Chia seeds - Grief

Hemp seeds - Sympathy

L-theanine - Compassion

Curcumin - Compassion

Resveratrol - Fair

Carrot seed oil - Tolerance

Dr. Miller's Holy Tea - Revitalization

Glucosamine Chondroitin Sulphate - Endowment

NOT SO SUPER SUPPLEMENTS
that fail to produce significant results.

Glutathione - glutathione is a protein synthesized in the liver from 3 amino acids; cystein, glycine and glutamine. It is essential to basic energy production in every cell of the body. It is a powerful anti-oxidant, neutralizes toxins and optimizes white blood cell functions. It supports the brain, the immune system and anti-aging. Glutathione is very poorly assimilated when administered orally as a supplement. Glutathione patches also do not live up to marketing claims. To boost levels of this important element use alpha lipoic acid, improve liver function and reduce toxic exposure. Raising glutathione levels is crucial for MS patients and Alzheimer's, but taking glutathione supplements will not provide the support needed for neurotransmitters and immune functions. It is effective when given intravenously.

Resveratrol - an extract concentrated from red grapes, this bioflavonoid is being marketed for anti-aging and immune support. The readings indicate that the red grapes are indeed very good for you but that this highly refined processed supplement does not provide anything near the benefit of its whole unprocessed food source - grapes.

Glucosamine and Chondroitin Sulfate - building blocks of cartilage, these elements are widely marketed together and with MSM as the cure for painful arthritis. The readings have never yet recommended this supplement for healing joints. Instead the readings recommend establishing normal pH and supplementing with essential fatty acids and a bone collegenizer such as Biosil by Natural Factors. Bone broth, and marrow broth, are full of these important elements in a bioavailable form that promotes healthy joints.

Curcumin - concentrated plant compounds from the spice tumeric is marketed as the cure for everything. Using it as a spice to create healthy food reads very high positive, but taking it as a supplement in capsules has never been recommended in the readings.

Acai - the whole berry, fresh or dried, is a powerhouse of antioxidants with benefits the same as blueberries and cherries. Processing it to make juice or capsules does not produce a substance of healing properties. Eating any locally sourced organic berries or cherries is a better choice than any form of acai imported from Brazil except whole fresh organic berries, which is equivalent but not better. Blueberries and cherries are cardio protective, anti-inflammatory and anti-cancer just as much as acai and more so in the case of processed refined products.

Kombucha - a fizzy fermented tea that, when fresh homemade, contains probiotics and enzymes to support digestive health. It is particularly beneficial for restoring balance in cases of chronic diarrhea and is specific for bowel infection with C-difficile (the most common cause of diarrhea in hospitals), because it contains the probiotic S.bulardii. The raw kombucha capsules and store bought kombucha drinks read anywhere from zero, neutral, safe to negative four point two. None of the bottled kombuchas is ever recommended in the readings.

Chia Seed - currently marketed as an excellent source of essential fatty acids and a vegan substitute for fish oil. Despite these marketing claims, chia seed does not read positive as a supplement, it reads -2.3. That means that chia seed does not metabolize in the human body the way these research models are projecting. They read as difficult to digest, metabolizing as only 20% protein and 30% sugar. Avocados are a much better source of both protein and essential fatty acids. Flax oil is a better neuro-nutrient for vegan sourced omegas.

Hemp Seed - marketed as a high protein, high fiber super food, hemp seeds read zero for human consumption in their natural form and negative in processed forms such as protein powders. For those who need a fiber supplement, Metamucil is a better choice.

Alkaline Water - drinking alkaline water does not alkalize the body. This premise that it could do so is based on a lack of insight into human physiology. Anything consumed by mouth goes directly to the stomach where the pH is and must be 5.3 because an acid pH is needed for the breakdown of food. Putting a water with high pH (of say 9) will require the consumption of salt (NaCl) to produce HCl or hydrochloric stomach acid to restore healthy pH to this part of the digestive system. What is needed is not food or water that is alkaline going in, but rather food that is alkalizing as it progresses through the digestive process. The functions of nutrient exchange and assimilation require an alkaline pH in the small intestine. The production of vitamins B, K and D require an alkaline pH in the large intestine as well. Drinking a structured water with a pH of about 5.3 to 5.5 is the best way to rehydrate and support optimum pH. Eating food that reacts with stomach acids and enzymes to produce alkaline pH can quickly restore healthy pH, but drinking alkaline water will only cause further disruption of the acid alkaline balance throughout the digestive system.

Coconut Oil - firmly established through marketing claims as a wonder food due to its MCT (medium chain triglycerides) content or its beneficial effects on cholesterol. Coconut oil has been questioned in hundreds of readings and attunements for clients and has never yet read positive for anyone. It reads -4.2 for internal use for humans because it is not easily metabolized and is stored in the liver, producing fatty liver. It does read positive for topical use on the skin (+6.4) and is nutritively beneficial when absorbed through the skin.

Liposomal Vitamin C - nature designed vitamin C to be a water soluble nutrient, such that normal physiology will concentrate this element in the kidney/adrenal complex, where it is most needed. Liposomal vitamin C has been designed by man to be fat soluble instead of water soluble, thus redirecting it away from its normal affinities and assimilation pathways. Rather than being an improvement, this designer nutrient reads at zero for benefiting the body. There is the potential negative consequence of believing one is supplementing with a high quality vitamin C when one is not effectively getting any support at all from this supplement.

SUSTAINABLE HEALTH EVERYDAY
First do no harm.

Hydrate - adults 10 cups of water daily, children age 3 and over about the same. To compensate for dehydration use Structured Water. Chronic sub-clinical dehydration is a leading health issue of our time.

Diet - 40% raw. Organic for the dirty dozen. Whole, fresh, local, in season. Less than 10% sugar. Avoid highly refined, processed foods: most bread, cookies, crackers, cereal, pasta, deli meats, processed cheese, junk food, ersatz food, cheese puffs, pork rinds, most chips, corn syrup, artificial sweeteners, rancid oils, canola oil, cotton seed oil. Failure to eliminate food, drug, and alcohol factors results in escalating toxic levels, chronic dehydration, falling vital force and weakened constitution. Eat healthy oils including olive oil. BLESS YOUR FOOD.

Avoid Prescription And Non Prescription Medicine - Reserve these for occasional use only and treat symptoms at their source by making naturally healthy choices.

Exercise - 60 minutes per day 6 days a week. Exercise is essential to support metabolism, peristalsis and circulation of the lymphatic system, and the production of CoQ10, the precursor to ATP (adenosine triphosphate) the basic energy unit of every cell.

Avoid Alcohol And Cigarettes - Eliminate these for a healing regime. The usual tolerance for alcohol is 3 servings per month of wine or beer and 2 per month of hard drinks, but not both. Tolerance for cigarettes varies from none to 3 to 6 per day but non-chemicalized brands such as American Spirit or Sherman's are preferable.

Avoid toxic exposure - pesticide, chemicals, chlorine, fluoride, mercury, lead, arsenic, cadmium, and thousands more.

Detox - elimination, colon cleanse, enemas, colonics, castor oil packs and baths. Lack of proper hydration together with sedentary habits and poor diet prevent proper elimination and produces a build-up of toxic burden in the body.

Rest - balance, relaxation, and silence are all necessary in the harmonious rhythm of a healthy life. Respect the need for repose as a component of resilience.

Happiness - learn to create a life that you want to live rather than make a living. Do more of what you love and what fills you with energy, enthusiasm, optimism and joy. Do not do what you hate or hate what you do and blame it on others.

Bodywork - Massage, Reflexology, Lymphatic Drainage, Osteopathic, Chiropractic. The body benefits greatly from the extra support of various kinds of body work to support healing and promote health.

Extra Support

Acidophilus, Reuteri, to fight yeast and support colon health.

Green Vibrance or Barley Green for detox, liver and blood.

Digestive Enzymes to support pancreas and duodenum.

Dr. Miller's Holy Tea to improve colon health.

Vitamin B Complex for stress and Folic Acid for brain.

CoQ10 for circulatory health, brain, oxygenation and energy.

Omega's - essential fatty acids and Flax seed oil - omega 3's.

Floradix - Nutritive tonics for recovery from chronic illness, anemia, malnutrition, broken bones, surgery.

Vitamin C for adrenal support and immune functions.

GSE - grapefruit seed extract, antibiotic, antiviral, anti-fungal - for immune support.

Oregano oil - for immune support, especially respiratory infections.

Quercetin - inhibits allergic symptoms including allergies due to leaky gut.

Lemon Juice - an alkalizer, kidney support, fights yeast.

Exclusion Diet - Eliminate: alcohol, over the counter drugs and prescriptions, artificial sweeteners, wheat, corn, soy, chicken, chocolate, orange juice, coffee, sugar and processed foods.

Elderberry Syrup or Colostrum for immune support.

Broth - 2 to 3 cups daily.

Fresh Ginger Tea - 3 to 5 cups daily.

Castor Oil Packs

Epsom Salts Baths or Kneipp Baths 1-800-937-4372.

Agave Sweetener or Melaluca honey

ProGest cream - hormonal support for peri-menopausal and menopausal women.

Emergen-C - for occasional use.

Rescue Remedy or other Bach Flower Remedies

Structured Water

Rest, naps, conscious relaxation

Exercise, yoga, walking

Massage, cranial adjustment

Emotional release work

Meditation, prayer, personal retreats, music

"This book is full of lists. The lists are suggested starting points for further research and study to discover which suggestions from each list are the best for each individual. Finding the best four to six recommendations from each list that most closely matches and best supports the needs of the individual, is the appropriate way to use the many lists of recommendations and suggestions found throughout this book. No person will ever need everything on any list."

Fravarti

ADDITIONAL SUPPORTIVE MEASURES
for acute illness.

1. Use **No Alcohol.** Alcohol both adds to the toxic burden and creates a hydration deficit which prevents further healing and detoxing until positive hydration can be re-established.

2. Both **prescriptions** and **OTC medications** are usually dehydrating and will need to be filtered from the body by the kidneys and liver. When medications are needed, be very conscientious about compensating for the physiological challenge by drinking copious amounts of water and consuming broth.

3. **Rescue Remedy** in water or directly into the mouth from the stock bottle or Rescue Remedy Pastilles, a non-alcohol formula in a soft lozenge can be used liberally. Any of these can be used continuously throughout the day or for many days as an extra support for your healing protocol.

4. **Penta Water** is a therapeutic grade of water that helps the body recover from dehydration and speeds the detoxing at both the cellular level as well as through the organs of elimination: lungs, kidneys, liver, colon, and skin. We live in a culture of dehydration and a pattern of chronic dehydration lies behind many illnesses and greatly hinders our ability to recover. Things that dehydrate us include High Fructose Corn Syrup, highly refined grains like bread, pasta, crackers, cookies, artificial sweeteners, over the counter medications, prescription medications, alcohol and coffee as well as caffeine in other forms.

5. Lower your **activity level** during acute illness. Seek balance and repose. Stay down and resist the temptations to fulfill expectations (your own or others) by continuing on with the scheduled activities. Withdraw into getting your own needs met at the level of the physical body or any other level at which you feel out of balance or unsupported.

6. Lower the **stress level.** Meditation and prayer are excellent ways to heal from the stress of life's challenges. Restore your faith that you are on the right track in the life you were meant to live, which is always full of potential in every moment. Make a commitment to pursue you own happiness and wellbeing relentlessly, but without the negative efforting of stress.

7. **Massage** in all forms: Lymphatic drainage, reflexology, deep tissue and neuro-muscular massage, as well as relaxing massage, are all significant supports for healing the physical body in times of both acute or chronic illness. Pain in the body can often be relieved by therapeutic massage.

8. **Soaking baths** including with Epsom salts, Sea salts or Dr. Kneipp therapeutic aromatherapy baths. (Kneippus.com or 1-800-937-4372 to order baths). Hydrotherapy and aromatherapy combine to provide a very effective therapeutic support for the recovering patient. One or more baths per day is often recommended. Hot tubs and jacuzzi's are also recommended for promoting relaxation and healing.

9. **Silence and Retreats** are both highly recommended for healing at all levels.

10. **Supplements** may include vitamins B and C, GSE, Oregano oil, Elderberry Syrup, herbal laxative (or enema), digestive enzymes and acidophilus.

11. Use food as medicine and **fasting** as needed to support recovery, especially from pneumonia or respiratory infection or stomach ailments. **High protein broth** is usually the food of choice to support a compromised patient. Eliminate all highly processed foods and eat only whole fresh food, preferably organic.

DETOXING THE BODY - WHEN, WHY, HOW

It is normal for the body to be continuously and effectively eliminating toxins through the actions of the many different organs and systems working together to optimize physiological conditions within the body. If the primary organs of detoxification and elimination become compromised, sluggish and inefficient, the toxic burden (the amount of toxins stored in the body) rises. When optimum pH (6.8) is maintained together with optimum hydration (through conscientious consumption of a pure diet and pursuit of an active lifestyle with a long-term focus on physical fitness) the body is able to efficiently detox and achieve sustainable health. In our American culture today, there are endemic toxins building up in the bodies of the population at large through repeated and habitual exposure to toxins which are not easily eliminated from the body. The cumulative exposure to toxins that undermine our health has been on the increase for 150 years as we have learned to use chemistry to create certain conveniences.

Since the advent of widespread use of GMO grains (American wheat, corn and soy) and foods (canola, HFCS and BT potatoes) in our industrialized food supply, the levels of routine exposure to bio-toxins has reached potentially lethal proportions.
The toxins of today's industrialized agriculture, which are in both our food and water supply, are gravely endangering all Americans who regularly consume processed foods, including: breads, pasta, cereal, crackers, cookies, pizza, chicken nuggets, french fries, all highly processed soy products and anything containing HFCS and or canola oil. These products today, unless certified organic, contain the toxin glyphosate (RoundUp) and are bio-engineered to tolerate this toxin. However, the human body (as well as those of our companion animals and our livestock) is not

bio-engineered to tolerate this poison.

Repeated exposure to this toxin results in an increasing accumulation of glyphosate in certain organs of the body. Of particular interest is its tendency to build up in the pituitary and the result is chemical castration, loss of desire, libido and function at the level of the brain. This is just one example, but a common one, of the thousands of ways bodies accumulate a toxic burden in our current culture.

There are two primary approaches to detoxing the body. One approach looks at things that can be done to the body or therapeutic modalities such as enemas, colonics, salt baths, castor oil packs, lymphatic drainage massage, sauna and exercise. The other focus is what one can take or eliminate in the form of supplements, food and drink.

Combining many different methods for supporting detoxification simultaneously is most effective. Certain methods are more effective for specific toxins and some methods are superior for generalized clearing of many non-specific toxins. Lowering the overall burden of stored toxins in the body can take many months, particularly because a high toxic reading is almost invariably accompanied by chronic dehydration (possibly sub-clinical) and acid or low pH, both of which must be corrected for the liver and kidneys to be able to do their jobs.

As to how to support lowering the toxic burden in the body, consumption is key. What to consume and what not to consume comes down to some very basic guidelines. Raw food is king and raw juice is high king - in both cases because it raises the pH (which takes the burden off the kidneys) and increases hydration - relative to eating cooked or processed foods. In most cases, three cups of raw juice daily will raise the body's pH to 6.8 in four weeks. Fasting and modified fasting (juice or broth) are the fastest way to restore balance, but can only be used for a short time and maybe only a few times a year, because they require a much lower level of activity for the duration of the fast, together with retreat like circumstances and state of mind. Fasting is not conducive to supporting engagement with mundania and it is highly recommended that one not just plan to go about one's normal daily routines or expectations while fasting. Juice fasting, particularly when supplemented with raw almond cream and possibly other raw foods such as avocado, can be maintained for weeks or even months, when the daily life routine and expectations are designed to support it. This is of great significance to those whose challenge is overcoming chronic disease (including cancer, Multiple Sclerosis, fibromyalgia and loss of cognitive function) when it is due to dehydration, acidosis and rising toxic levels, as is the case with many dementias. For the purpose of detoxing, a diet that is 80% to 100% raw is recommended. Once the body has recovered a state of health and well being, a maintenance diet of 40% to 60% raw food will be sufficient in most cases.

Additional ways to support detoxing the body through conscious consumption includes the option of drinking lemon water. Edgar Cayce recommended 8 oz. of lemon water 8 times a day made from the juice of 1/2 fresh lemon in 8 oz. water. This is a slow gentle kidney cleanse and is best to continue for many months. There are also many botanicals and herbal formulas which are effective in supporting the body in its continual mandate to purify and detoxify. One of the most famous of such formulas is Essiac which, together with its sister formula Flor-Essence, well deserves its reputation as an anti-cancer and cancer preventative tonic or tea. Herbal bitters formulas and herbal colon cleanses, as well as anti-parasitic herbs (such as black walnut and wormwood) are all useful for supporting a digestive system cleanse, but should be used with care and guidance as to amount, duration, frequency and compatibility with the needs of the individual.

Conscious consumption for the purpose of detoxing and healing the body also requires conscious elimination of many common toxins that are a routine part of our cultural consumption heritage. It means not eating what other people may be eating or feel entitled to eat, because doing so is in direct conflict with goals for immediate and long term well-being. Among the most frequently recommended items to eliminate include all processed foods as they are usually old, depleted or devoid of significant food value.

They are suppressive to the normal physiological functions such as the balance of the appetite hormone leptin, due to the presence of such GMO factors as HFCS, canola and cottonseed oil, and wheat, corn and soy. These convenience foods or food substitutes are the greatest contributor to a chronic and persistent weakening of the body due to increasing acidosis and concurrent dehydration. Eating these processed foods can increase the body's need for water from 8 cups per day to 18 cups per day - an amount which one can not realistically drink and thus a water debt sets in from this cycle of water deficit. Once there is a water debt established in the body (dehydration), the physiological processes of the liver, kidneys, adrenals, lymphatic system, heart, thyroid, and even bones and brain are all compromised, and reduced in their effectiveness and efficiency in sustaining health. The toxic burden in the body begins to escalate as more toxins are going into the system than are being eliminated. Some of these toxins will be stored in fat cells, some in the bones, and some will have affinity to accumulate in specific organs and systems. Once the physiological process of storing the excess toxins in the body has begun, it is wise to implement as many different ways of restoring health and balance as may be warranted, changing from doing what seems convenient to doing what really works to create the best health.

Much of the toxic burden in the body enters through the gut. One of the most important supplements to support health in the gut is probiotics. For the upper digestive and illeum, lactobacilis and bifidus are specific and for the lower digestive and the colon reuteri is necessary. The probiotic reuteri is beneficial for clearing candida overgrowth (yeast), arsenic and the GMO toxin glyphosate, which is widely present throughout the American food supply.

Signs or indications that the body would benefit from a focus on detoxifying can include any or almost all of the following signs of toxicity: anxiety, anger, chronic frustration or confusion, irritability, depression, cognitive problems, memory, Alzheimer's, chronic fatigue, sluggish liver, inability to digest, especially fats, indigestion, bloating, gas, colic, heartburn, bad taste in the mouth, bad breath and body odor (including foot odor), constipation, allergies to foods, drugs, fragrances and cleaning agents, overweight, poor immunity, sinus infections, edema (swelling) including around the eyes, face, fingers, feet, legs and belly, hangover feeling, headaches, vertigo, pain, inflammation, numbness, tingling, lethargy, generalized weakness, skin dry, flaky, cracked, rashes, eczema, psoriasis, hives, acne, rosacea, boils, cardiovascular disease, hypertension, cancer, MS, fibromyalgia and type 2 diabetes.

Methods Or Treatments For Detoxing

Fasting - (on water) or modified fasting (raw juice, broth or ginger tea) Hannah Kroger's 5 day watermelon fast for kidney detox.

Elimination diet - eliminate processed grains including wheat, corn and soy, whole meats (broth is allowed), chocolate, alcohol, HFCS, artificial sweeteners, industrial grade (non-organic) dairy (in some cases organic dairy may be used), sugar, coffee, caffeine, seafood, roasted nuts and heated or rancid oils in general, chemicals and preservatives.

Eat whole fresh foods - especially raw, especially greens, organic if possible.

Hydration - 12 cups of water per day, structured water is better, Penta is best.

Enemas and colonics - including plain water enemas, 4 oz. of flax oil added to water, herbal infusions including chaparral, coffee enemas, and possible reuteri implant at the end of colon hydrotherapy to help reduce yeast overgrowth.

Herbal cleanses - including Colon Cleanse, Essiac and Flor-Essence, Dr. Miller's Holy Tea.

Edgar Cayce castor oil packs - over liver, omentum and painful joints (arthritis).

Fiber - such as ground flax seed and bentonite clay (Sonne's #7) or Zeolite.

Tinctures - including black walnut, wormwood, bupleurum, burdock, yellow dock, ginger, watermelon seed tea.

Bowel flora/probiotics - reuteri, lactobacillis, and bifidis.

Exercise - 60 to 90 minutes daily to detox liver, kidneys and lymphatics.

Chelation - with: DMPS, oral Calcium EDTA, I.V. Calcium EDTA, I.V. Vitamin C or Detoxamin suppositories.

Dry brushing - together with salt baths and salt scrubs, baking soda and herbs. Heat from the bath stimulates vasodilation and supports detoxing. Sauna is particularly important for detoxing organophosphates (such as the fertilizer Atrazine).

Oral health - dental cleanings, GSE in water.

Meditation - prayer, music or other spiritual practice to replace stress reactions and toxic thoughts.

Targeting Specific Organs Or Systems

Liver detox and fat detox - Exercise, weight loss, elimination diet, fasting and modified fasting, castor oil packs, alpha lipoic acid, Essiac, 80% raw food diet.

Bowel detox - Oral calcium EDTA, exercise, weight loss, probiotics - particularly reuteri, digestive enzymes, ginger tea, colonics and enemas, flax seed, Detoxamin suppositories, castor oil packs, wheatgrass juice, Barley Green or Green Vibrance, burdock root, GSE, Paragone, Candidagone and Candida Quick Cleanse.

Kidney detox - structured water especially Penta water, lemon juice in 8 oz water 8 x a day, watermelon fast, zeolite, Flor-Essence, oral calcium EDTA, raw juice to raise pH.

Lymph detox - Essential fatty acids, flax oil, evening primrose oil, Vitamin C, 100% raw food diet, watermelon seed tea, kombucha, cordyceps mushrooms, trampoline, sauna, massage, dry brushing, eucalyptus bath, intravenous Vitamin C, Essiac, GSE.

Blood detox - structured water, especially Penta water, intravenous Vitamin C, N-acetyl cysteine (must clear any yeast overgrowth before beginning NAC), Oregano Oil, beets, pycnogenols, Kneipp Juniper bath, hyperbaric oxygen.

Bone detox - MSM, fish oils, castor oil packs, Detoxamin suppositories, DMPS, 100% raw food diet, raw calcium.

Brain detox - structured water, especially Penta water, Acetyl L-carnitine, 100% raw food diet, hyperbaric oxygen, fish oils, raw almond cream, NAC.

Targeting Specific Toxins

Aluminum - the EPA threshold of 50 ppb reads as equalling +4.3 toxic reading. Accumulates in the brain and nervous system and drinks in aluminum cans are considered to be a culpable source. Drink beer and sodas from glass bottles only. Chelate out aluminum with oral calcium EDTA.

Mercury - the EPA threshold of 5.8 micrograms per liter reads as equalling +3.2 toxic reading. Mercury accumulates in the brain and liver and binds to cells including neurons. Chelate out mercury with calcium EDTA, Detoxamin or DMSA.

Cadmium - is of particular interest in the American Northwest where cadmium exposure is common and profoundly affects dental health. Chelate out cadmium with DMPS, or acetyl L-carnitine and homeopathy.

Arsenic - use reuteri and oral calcium EDTA to chelate out arsenic.

Fluoride - Detoxamin suppositories and castor oil packs especially for bones.

Lead - DMPS, I.V. glutathione and zeolite.

Flame retardants - calcium EDTA.

BT - pesticide toxin from GMO potatoes, American french fries are made from these - use calcium EDTA and Udo's Super 8 probiotics

Carbomates - pesticides such as Raid and Black Flag - Vitamin C and calcium EDTA

Organophosphates - industrial fertilizer such as Atrazine use calcium EDTA, raw juice, sauna.

Carbon Monoxide - Hyperbaric Oxygen

Radiation - radium, uranium, polonium, strontium 90 - use raw juice and intravenous calcium EDTA or intravenous vitamin C.

Chelation of glyphosate - (RoundUp) from specific organs and systems pituitary - use homeopathy, consider DMPS, hyperbaric oxygen.

prostate - homeopathy (sepia)

blood - wheatgrass juice, hyperbaric oxygen.

lymph nodes - raw juice, homeopathy, Flor-Essence, castor oil packs.

kidneys – calcium EDTA, magnesium.

intestines - reuteri, lactobaccillis and bifidis, raw juice, Flor-Essence, Green Vibrance.

The following cannot currently be effectively chelated out of the body: use hyperbaric oxygen therapy.

Phthalates - source shampoo, deodorant, lotions and soap, soft plastics.

Perfluro octanoic acids - source teflon.

PCB's - polychlorinated biphenols.

DDT - pesticide.

Dioxins - Agent Orange, Round up.

Clearing toxins from the body is a slow, molecule by molecule process. It takes much longer than we expect even with the support of homeopathy and well chosen supplements. Both steroids and statins (cholesterol drugs) take about one year per month of prescription medication to clear all its residues from the body. Barbiturates like Phenobarbitol and Seconal, as well as pain blockers, like morphine and OxyContin, each take about a year to clear fifteen doses. Some toxins are cumulative and the body does not eliminate them effectively, or at all, without a chelating agent to bind to the toxin and move it out.

STRESS AND CORTISOL

During my attunements for clients, I frequently check how they are reading for stress on a 10 point scale. The amount of physical stress that reads beneficial for the human body is +2.4 which is the equivalent to the stress of a healthy baby learning to crawl and to walk. The average adult in America is trying to function at their best while enduring a stress level that reads +4.4 which is far enough beyond the optimum as to become detrimental if maintained overlong. Physical stress is composed of effort, nutritional demands, hydration, sleep, environmental factors (including temperature and sound levels) and physiology, including pH. Optimum psychological stress is also +2.4 and reflects a level of stress that holds our interests and keeps us alert, aware, consciously present and confident. The average adult in America today reads for a persistent psychological stress level of +4.4 due to factors in the outlook that include fear, grief, worry, depression, relationship, self image, money issues, health concerns and the control dramas that these can evoke.

Both of these forms of stress raise cortisol levels preparing the body for fight or flight. Whether defending against the perceived threat of unjust criticism or the threat of survival itself, these forms of stress keep us edgy, as if something overwhelming is happening or is about to happen. That edgy feeling is often accompanied by feelings of nausea and sometimes vertigo together with restlessness, as if you have to do something and yet are aware of being tired, depleted. We use our determination and will power to endure through persistent high stress as a cultural value signifying worthiness of success through our personal sacrifice and diligence. We try harder, but we don't always try smarter. Culturally, we feel it is smart to endure high levels of stress for as long as possible. The physical body, however, needs its stress experiences to be in the form of interval training, a balance of activity and repose, a balance of concern with unconcern.

The body needs its Sabbath in order to be sustained by the continuous healing rejuvenation of the body that never stops. If we use up more of the body's energy, sustenance and resilience than it has, there needs to be reparation - a time for the Divine physician to repair the body and restore its full capacities. If this responsibility to nurture one's strength and resilience through a sustainable balance of the body's real needs is ignored, then a deficit sets in resulting in a depletion of vitality, a depletion of coping skills on all levels including personality and cognitive function.

Reparation in the form of meditation, yoga, massage, retreats, silence, juice fasts, journaling or self-nurturing are all necessary because our lives contain such extremes of stress both circumstantially (struggles over freedom, relationship, loss, money) and skyrocketing levels of environmental stress (noise, chemicals, food) that extra healing support is needed on a very regular basis, in fact, daily. We need a little bit of Sabbath in every day and some days we need a lot.

In America today, we are maintaining cortisol levels that average 25% higher than is optimum for the body to maintain sustainable health. Chronic high cortisol levels trigger biochemical mechanisms which cause damage in the hippocampus in the brain due to the very high number of cortisol receptors in the brain which bind cortisol to that site causing the destruction of neurons and brain atrophy. Prolonged grief, depression, PTSD and emotional distress impairs cognitive functions and memory because the hippocampal neurons are binding cortisol.

We need to lower our cortisol levels consciously and regularly throughout every day. There are dozens of ways to lower cortisol intentionally if we are aware of the desire to do so, but they all take time, attention and resources so we have to be highly motivated and present to the need to lower cortisol. In some ways, cortisol is all about presence, about who you show up as: stressed or calm and clear, agitated or relaxed, anxious and over controlling or confident and tolerant. The self concept in every moment is directly linked to raising and lowering the cortisol levels.

Cortisol flooding uses up enormous amounts of hydration, specifically, to protect the neurons in the brain which are vulnerable to burning up when cortisol levels are high. Chronic subclinical dehydration and low or acidic pH result in physiological stress that elevates cortisol levels even more than psychological stress or physical effort. Chronic stress levels that produce cortisol levels persistently averaging 125% of normal optimal cortisol levels in the body will burn up an additional 6 cups of hydration daily. This additional requirement of hydration is signaled to the brain as anxiety and the first and leading symptom of dehydration is anxiety. Rehydrating dramatically lowers cortisol levels and protects the brain, kidneys, heart and adrenals immediately and it relieves anxiety.

Years of dehydration, acidosis and cortisol flooding disrupt the acetyl choline cycle of the brain and diminish cognitive function and memory. This is the primary cause of Alzheimer's type dementia. To protect the brain from cortisol flooding and support cognitive function the choice to consider, second only to hydration in its protective capacity, is CoQ10 or co-enzyme Q10. Every cell of the body needs CoQ10 as it is the precursor to the basic form of energy for the cell - ATP, short for adenosine triphosphate. The body makes its own CoQ10 but only if you exercise. Liver health is also integral to the body's ability to manufacture CoQ10 in amounts sufficient to serve the needs of every cell of the body. Many prescription medications, including statins to lower cholesterol, severely deplete the body of CoQ10.

Chronic stress, whether physical or psychological, and the resultant levels of elevated cortisol in the body, also will ultimately result in lower progesterone levels, particularly in peri-menopausal and post-menopausal women because the hormone precursor (they use the same one) is all going into the production of extra cortisol. Use of progesterone cream and supplementation with pregnenalone (it's precursor) are among the first considerations for extra support. The other source of safe natural progesterone is raw fruits and vegetables, and it is especially concentrated in raw juice. It is not possible to get too much progesterone or hurt yourself with it because when all progesterone receptors are filled, progesterone converts to other hormones the body needs including estrogen and cortisol.

How To Lower Cortisol

Drink water - if even slightly dehydrated, drink 1 liter of structured water. Add Rescue Remedy, 6 droppers full, per 1 liter of structured water, and/or use Rescue Remedy Pastilles.

Protein - Eat high quality protein three times a day, in forms the body most readily assimilates - including broths, eggs, raw nuts and seeds, raw nut creams and fresh homemade nut milks and avoiding processed meats and processed milks (both dairy and non-dairy). Consuming 30 to 32% of calories as protein can lower cortisol up to 15%.

Raw juice - Daily raw juice will lower cortisol by about 15%, in part by improving pH and hydration. Keeping the pH at 6.6 to 6.9 will lower cortisol by up to 20% by taking the burden off the kidneys.

Take a nap - Catch up on sleep. Convince the adrenals that you are lying in a hammock sipping lemonade and they are not needed.

Take a bath - Soak in a hot tub, take a shower or go swimming. 20 minutes in water completely changes the aura and sense of well-being.

Conscious relaxation - Yoga, exercise that is gently centered in the body.

Meditation - Prayer, solitude, alone time, journaling.

Creative time - Arts, poetry, crafts.

Listen to music - Play music. Dance. Fun and games, non-competitive play.

Massage - Foot rubs, back rubs, hugs, cuddles, positive touch.

Clean/organize.

Make to do lists - Lots of lists, as long as you like. List making lowers cortisol.

Chewing gum - Lowers cortisol, especially if you are trying to quit smoking. Choose a brand that has benefits for oral health like Peelu or Spry.

Avoid alcohol - High Fructose Corn Syrup, rancid oils and GMO grains and GMO oils

Medications - Avoid over the counter and prescription medications.

Reduce processed - foods to less than 20% of diet.

Observe "Alarmist" thinking - and reprogram for non-crisis outlook and response. Yes, talk yourself out of being crazy and put a positive spin on your version of reality. Affirm safety and security in the present moment.

Reduce "efforting" - don't try too hard, don't over-do. Strive for excellence, not perfection. Go with the flow. Don't over plan. Be flexible.

Reduce activity levels - Do few things but do them well. Choose activities that leave you feeling uplifted, optimistic, enthusiastic and restored.

Balance activity with repose - Through out each day and through the weeks.

Stop your expectations - of yourself and others and how you think it should be - and for just one hour - let it be. Don't forsake your goals. Just take a break, catch your breath and find your happy thought. Happiness creates health.

Live slowly - eat slowly, talk slowly, and do each as if you were going to live forever, and enjoy the process of everything you choose to do and of everything life requires of you. Make an art of handling all challenges as beautifully as possible.

Remember, you can't get it wrong - There is a department of getting all things right in the Universe - and you're not it. The Creator and Sustainer never put the divine perfection into the hands of limited imperfect beings. Things are still alright and you're doing fine.

Nobody else is getting it wrong either - Relent of your judgments and criticisms. "Neither do I condemn you" Christ said, as our exemplar.

Balance the budget and live realistically - Be practical. Do what works.

When we respond to the stresses of modern life as if everyday irritations and challenges were life threatening, the resultant chronic cortisol flooding destroys neurons in the brain and interferes with the consolidation of memory and cognitive functions. It also causes the adrenals to release catacholomines into the bloodstream which damage the heart muscle and decreases the body's normal immune response, decreasing DNA repair which can contribute to cancer and increasing hyper auto immune reactions and diseases such as MS and Lupus. Our perception and interpretation of our challenges determines whether they contribute the damaging effects in the body that are the outcome of prolonged extreme stress. Developing good coping skills and a positive psychological outlook supports health and healing. We can learn to modify our outlook and reactions to support happiness.

In America, the average stress reading on men, women and children over age five is about +4.2. An optimal reading on stress levels in human physiology is 2.2 to 2.5. The higher than optimal physiological stress level in the body is due to three main factors. When the stress level is high and increasing there is always a challenge in the lymphatic system. The reason behind it in America most often is diet and the continuous exposure to glyphosate and other industrial food toxins. The next most significant influence after industrial food toxins is prescription medicines. When diet and medications produce dehydration - even subclinical dehydration, the stress on the kidneys is increased exponentially. Acid pH below the normal range for human physiology is the number one greatest challenge to normal kidney function. The burden on the kidneys increases 100% for each three tenths of a point below the normal pH of 6.7. This is because it is the kidneys job to keep the blood pH at 7.364 to 7.365. A blood pH of 7.4 is usually fatal and is an indication of kidney failure.

The third and most obvious factor affecting the stress reading is happiness. A high positive happiness reading corresponds to lower physiological stress and a zero or negative happiness reading corresponds to a higher physiological stress in the body. When psychological challenges resolve physiologic stress improves also. Americans tend to choose a high stress life style for themselves and their children because of their cultural conditioning that their success in life depends on placing high value on doing as much as humanly possible each day and sometimes more. I call this the push of the cultural paradigm to catch up as part of the formula for success.

However, doing as much as one can do every day will result in physical and psychological depletion; feeling used up for one's long term goals and larger projects. It is important not to use use up one's vitality each day but rather to cultivate a reserve of energy, activity and repose.

SLEEP, REST, RELAXATION, REPOSE

Currently in America, recently published statistics indicate that 56 million prescriptions per year are written for sleep medications. We are among the most sleep deprived cultures ever to evolve. In part, this is because we have cultivated staying busy as a coping mechanism, a psychological defense to support our avoidance of what we don't want to look at, feel or deal with. We habitually seek validation of our essential self-worth through our relentless pursuit of doing and particularly of doing all that we can to the point of doing too much, until it breaks us. Reaching this breaking point through over doing is necessary to the ego trying to see itself as good enough and having proof that one has done all that is possible is one of our benchmarks of goodness. Being perpetually too busy is a common way of avoiding the discomfort that can come in a quiet moment of awareness that one is doing many things that are diminishing one's happiness rather than enhancing it. In this regard, of doing and not doing, we can be very poor judges of what will create happiness.

Leading causes of chronic sleeplessness in our time can be categorized as three basic types, each of which has its own solutions. All three of these sources of insomnia can be concurrently present in one individual. Frequently, long term sleeplessness is a manifestation of adrenal weakness. This type of sleep deprivation accompanies states of physical and emotional overwhelm that arise from the habit of expecting too much, doing too much, perfectionism and a critical, judgmental outlook, trauma, stress, anxiety, and mental/emotional illnesses such as bi-polar disorder and PTSD.

Sleep disruption produces depression. This happens because sleep is essential to brain processing and memory consolidation. Sleep deprivation inhibits the body's regenerative functions and promotes both insulin resistance and weight gain. Lack of sleep and dysregulated sleep also produce poor judgement, impulsiveness, poor memory and concentration and a craving for stimulants, especially sugar and caffeine.

The second common source of severely impaired sleep pattern is the thyroid/brain connection which is a weakness that results from acid pH of 5.7 or below, which is a full point below normal and this state of acidosis produces a disruption of the acetyl choline cycle of the brain, increasing insulin resistance and slowing metabolism, often in conjunction with weight gain or obesity and concurrent malnutrition. This type of insomnia is a disease of consumption and can be caused by prescription medications, especially those used continuously for years, together with a diet of highly refined and processed convenience foods.

The third common source of inability to sleep is hormone imbalance. This includes low progesterone just before and during the menses, even lower progesterone during and after menopause and chronic cortisol flooding which uses up the hormone precursors and thus depletes the progesterone level secondarily. Progesterone is a sleep hormone. In this category also include sleeplessness due to iron anemia or malnutrition, both of which can cause restless leg syndrome.

Among the successful modalities of natural support for restoring healthy sleep cycles, there are important daily lifestyle choices: physical fitness/exercise, stress reduction/balance and a wholesome diet of fresh fruit and vegetables and raw juice to raise the pH and heal the adrenals. Conscious stress reduction is a healthy habit to cultivate. Practice relaxation, rest, repose, silence or quiet time every day, lowering the activity level by 20%, prioritize and rebalance the schedule for more down time, restful activities and practice stillness. Learn to do nothing and call it Zen time, the art of being.

Journaling and writing to do lists are also habits that help us decompress. These two simple things tend to get things off our minds so we don't have to keep going over things and reimpressing ourselves with our version of our story or reminding ourselves of what we are afraid we may forget. We can let it go or we can change it once we feel we really have the insight we needed from telling our story the way we did. Breathing practices, meditation and centering prayer also help to nourish an empowering outlook by reminding us that we are more than we appear to be and that there is a greater power than ourselves continually creating harmony and perfection in the Universe and that we are always connected to that greater power as well as to all of creation.

When simply doing less and cultivating balanced restful activities isn't enough or doesn't seem to be a real option, it may be time to find a good counselor. Cognitive behavior therapy, in particular, helps one retrain both conditioned thinking and habits to better support personal goals for health and wellbeing through new positive programming.

Good psychological health alone may not be enough to restore healthy sleep patterns if there is a significant metabolic disturbance, as is the case with weakening thyroid function in conjunction with disruption of the acetylcholine cycle of the brain due to chronic acidosis (acid pH) and dehydration. This metabolic weakness often presents with both obesity and malnutrition and frequently includes a long history of multiple prescription medications over a period of years for a variety of ever increasing physical and psychological challenges.

Poor health produces a poor quality of sleep. A comprehensive healing protocol would include raw juice daily to raise the pH, increasing raw food in general and adding high protein broth where necessary to raise the dietary intake of protein to 30 to 32% of total consumption. This easily assimilated form of protein helps lower cortisol levels, increases strength and resilience, and supports metabolic balance and rehydration. In addition to the necessary changes in diet and medications, this particular type of sleep disturbance responds particularly well to increased levels of exercise and physical fitness which helps to reset the metabolism.

For chronic insomnia due to metabolic imbalances, 90 minutes of exercise daily is recommended. In fact, for all types of insomnia, increasing exercise to this level has better results for 90% of people than any other single method known. Yoga, Tai Chi and Chi Gong can be even more beneficial than some other forms of exercise because of the emphasis on conscious awareness of personal energy, space, and balance and deliberate intentional healthy embodiedness harmonizing inner and outer, spiritual and mundane.

In addition to lowering stress levels, raising physical fitness and optimizing diet, there are many more choices that may provide some immediate though possibly temporary support. A thirty minute warm bath or soak in a hot tub helps the body and mind relax and often produces drowsiness. The body will respond to the warm soak by moving heat out of the core to the extremities which is conducive to sleep. Adding a couple of cups of Epsom Salts to the warm water is also helpful because the magnesium in it can be absorbed through the skin and helps regulate the serotonin levels in the brain.

Aromatherapy added to the bath is also a significant therapeutic support. Dr. Kneipp's deep sleep bath formula of Valerian & Hops is safe and effective and very calming, even for children. Lavender baths and linen sachets are historically renown for this purpose as well.

Certain widely available natural supplements also have a proven history when it comes to promoting and prolonging sleep. A night time combination of 1 gram of calcium plus 1 gram of magnesium taken together with 5 mgs of melatonin to support the pineal gland in the brain has a track record of providing noticeable improvement when taken 2 hours before bed. When chronic sleeplessness is manifesting along with chronic states of high anxiety or trauma, a supplement of 5HTP may be effective in supporting higher levels of serotonin. A supplement of CoQ10 may also help sleep patterns by improving circulation, oxygenation and protecting the neurons in the brain from excess cortisol.

For women, and more than twice as many women are affected by lack of sleep than men, a supplement of progesterone cream applied daily for many months can help to restore a healthy sleep cycle as well as make stronger, healthier bones and younger looking skin. After menopause, a woman's only source of progesterone other than supplements is raw fruits and vegetables, especially raw juice.

Avoiding alcohol is the best choice when facing a sleep deficit as drinking alcohol produces a poor quality of sleep and the body tends to awaken at about 3am due to the other physiological consequences on the liver, kidneys, brain and nervous system. Combining alcohol with prescription or over the counter sleep medications is unwise and is the most common source of strange and unusual side effects including sleep walking and sleep eating.

Bodywork, including reflexology (feet) and neuro-muscular (deep trigger point) massage as well as osteopathic adjustments can all help to promote a deeper rest and more refreshing sleep. This type of physical therapy not only supports the healing of physical pain and limitations, it also significantly improves mental/emotional health and lowers psychological stress and helps the individual release and transform on several integrated levels at once creating an experiential foundation for periods of profound well-being.

A master homeopath can provide additional support for recovery of healthy sleep cycles through careful use of homeopathic remedies including possibly Staphysagria, Nux Vomica, Nat. Mur., or Sepia depending on the exact presentation of symptoms and the personality and reactions of the sleep deprived individual. Also Bach Flower remedies may promote sleep through better emotional balance and stability. In particular Red Chestnut for being plagued with worries and anxiety or choose Star of Bethlehem for trauma and shock and Gentian for persistent self-doubt. The Bach Flower remedies can be used in combinations when more than one seems to match the circumstances and the best carrier for these flower remedies is to put them in structured water and sip them throughout the day, usually for a few weeks.

Lastly, but of great importance, the ambience of the bedroom can be optimized to improve quality and duration of sleep. A clean room, free of clutter, calms the mind and nervous system. An environment free of dust, dirt and pet dander makes it easier to breathe deeply and the better breathing relaxes the body more deeply. A comfortable mattress with just the right pillows, appealingly soft fresh bedcovers in attractive colors, clean sheets and smells everywhere, fresh air and sufficient darkness, can all make a difference in the quest for a great night's sleep. Lowering the room temperature to just below 70 degrees encourages snuggling into the covers and is more conducive to sleep than a warm room. Silence is an excellent support for high quality sleep but when silence is not an option, choose either relaxing music, white noise like a fan or nature sounds like rain or ocean waves. A habit of using familiar calming sounds regularly is also an inducement to relaxing into sleep.

For those who are taking all possible steps to balance their sleep cycles but are currently somewhere in the process and can't go to sleep right now, tonight, or can't go back to sleep, it is often best to get out of bed and do something else for an hour or two until sleepiness begins to set in, as it ultimately will. Plan for quiet relaxing nighttime activities including writing in your journal about what's on your mind that's keeping you up at night, reading or taking a bath, meditation, prayer and other spiritual practices.

Avoid late night texting, internet and television as they are stimulating and unlikely to help you get enough good quality sleep if you are operating on a deficit. Sleep flexible hours when necessary and planning for naps during the day when feeling tired would be prudent. Relax your expectations. Sleep when you're sleepy and sleep when you can. Sleep, rest and repose are a strong foundation for balance, strength and stability. Trying to push on through with one's expectations (or other's) when experiencing sleep deficit is an accident waiting to happen.

EXERCISE AND SUSTAINABLE HEALTH

The need for exercise to keep the human body healthy is an adamant part of our collective cultural outlook. We all agree that it is important for sustainable health, strength and resilience to be physically fit and physical fitness activities abound in our culture. Walking, running, tennis, bicycling, skating, yoga, pilates, trampoline, weights, martial arts, dance, hula hoops and many, many more options are widely available and culturally encouraged. Even so, some people exercise and some people don't. Those who don't will have reasons for their choice - why they don't... but the outcome of not exercising is no respecter of good reasons.

The health of the liver, kidneys, adrenals, heart, thyroid and lymphatic system are all intrinsically tied to the level of physical activity. Exercise can lower cortisol levels which supports heart, adrenal, kidneys and nervous system health. Exercise improves circulation of blood and heart health and also improves circulation of lymph and immune health and supports detoxing the body. Exercise improves stamina and resilience to get through what each day requires of you and then it helps you sleep longer, deeper and more restfully. Both the exercise and the extra sleep it induces are good for metabolism and thyroid health and help promote weight loss and hormone balance. Exercise increases over all confidence, optimism and enthusiasm in one's outlook and is a source of strength in overcoming frustrations and depression. It improves mental and emotional health just as profoundly as it does physical health.

Being in touch with the body and it's real needs includes, over the long term, an average of two hours of physical exercise oriented activities per day. This is considerably more than the widely heard suggestions that one hour three times a week is sufficient. It might be enough, if you're young enough, if you're already strong enough and if you're healthy, but if we are looking at exercise for recovery of health and anti-aging benefits, then the truth is, that more than an hour a day is necessary for optimal results and two to three hours a day several times a week, even everyday when possible, works best. This is a lot of time, a major focus of energy and concentration of time, so make it a physical activity you love. Being happy during exercise and physical activities influences one to use more energy, work deeper and get better results.

Holding the concentration of a yoga practice for 30 years can result in a body that is 20 years younger than the cultural standard for their age and the same is true for other forms of physical mastery. If we want an anti-aging miracle, a fountain of youth that cannot be taken away from us, regular exercise is one of three essential elements to support that goal.

Taking an interest in and developing the body's ability to stretch, to move and to balance are innate from birth. A baby never stops moving, never stops exercising and deliberately pursuing the development of physical abilities. Some people are more kinesthetic than others and move much more freely and easily in their body than the cultural average. Other people feel more naturally oriented to the happy as a clam to stay in one spot outlook, maybe experiencing an active inner life of creative imagination in a sedentary body. It is also a choice, an identity or self concept that one takes on and defines oneself as a certain self image associated with a certain level of physical strength and ability relative to who you are willing to see yourself as. Who you conceive yourself to be changes very quickly when physical strength, stamina and resilience allow you to optimize your possibilities. If you are physically strong and of greater abilities, you are able to enjoy more of what life is continually offering you. Staying physically fit is one of the best, wisest, long term choices anyone can make.

Learning specifically to exercise and strengthen one's core is especially important for one's immune system. Not only is 70% of the immune system in the gut but so too do we hold our identity in the gut, our self image. If our self concept says we have a strong core then it supports us quite reliably and we tend to experience less self doubt and more confidence, courage even. It is important to choose exercise that specifically supports you in overcoming your physical weaknesses. This means you need to know yourself and your strengths, weaknesses and limitations and your current balance, rhythm and timing in your life. Some periods are very conducive to a build up of physical activities and exercise. At other times, life puts you on retreat and demands a lower level of activity to support rebuilding through rest, repose and balance. Finding exactly the right combination of exercise and repose for you is a matter of paying attention daily, staying interested in the real needs of the body so that it can serve you better and being more responsible than rebellious in relation to what really is sustainable in the human body.

Physical fitness constitutes a greater percentage of our health, well-being and functional capacity than we tend to think. If you're in good health, then about 1/3 of your health is dependent upon your maintaining physical fitness. If you are in need of recovering your health, then it is about 60% of your recovery that is dependent upon attaining physical fitness. Choosing not to exercise is choosing not to fully recover and not to be your best, most capable self. This is a choice that begins with your identity, your chosen and adapted self concept. Who are you choosing to be? Choosing greater physical health is a choice which supports creating more happiness. You can upgrade your choice of how to see yourself to one which suits you more perfectly today.

"To be in an environment that gives you joy, where every step you take awakens enjoyment, where you see the sunlight dappling through the trees, see the colors and smell the fragrance of the flowers, this is what makes you well".

Rudolph Steiner

BRAIN

Everything we feel, think, see, say and do is dependent upon brain function. We can take responsibility for sustainable brain health and thereby empower ourselves beyond all measure. The adult brain has approximately the same number of neurons as there are galaxies in the universe. When these neurons are activated, or fire, the electrochemical message of the neurotransmitters lights up the landscape of the brain like complex structures of tens of thousands of stars.

Normal aging is not associated with major cognitive decline, and yet in our time, it is becoming common place, such that more than half those who live past 85 years of age will manifest some form of senile dementia. Neuroscience of our day says this is due to lifestyle choices, and many factors which influence it are under our control. Risk factors for brain health which increase the likelihood of age related loss of cognitive function include: head injuries (sports), high sugar diet, obesity, elevated cholesterol, diabetes, hypertension, atherosclerosis, stroke, smoking, long history of anti-depressant medications, large number of intercurrent prescriptions for a period of years, chronic stress, and hormone replacement in women over age 65. Any diagnosis of Mild Cognitive Impairment (MCI) has an 85% likelihood of progressing to dementia, particularly Alzheimer's disease.

Factors that significantly decrease risk and support brain health include: maintaining normal weight, avoiding obesity and diabetes, regular consumption of large amounts of raw fruits and vegetables (especially raw juice), omega 3 essential fatty acids such as salmon and raw almond cream, exercise because it increases mitosis in the hippocampus producing new neurons. Also, continuing intellectual challenge, learning new things, social bonds to family and loved ones keeps oxytocin flowing. Learning to intentionally lower stress stops cortisol binding in the hippocampus thus preventing neural damage and brain atrophy which are seen in Alzheimer's brains.

Brain injuries, lesions and diseases often result in personality changes as they have a profound effect on the self concept through the body/mind feedback loops. Atrophy (shrinkage) of the hippocampal area of the mid-brain caused by the binding of cortisol appears in the brains of adults who were abused as children, those who experience prolonged grief or depression, PTSD or any long term extreme distress. This impairs cognitive function and memory.

Degenerative Brain Diseases

Current research with MRI's have shown the brains of dementia patients, including Alzheimer's, to be much reduced in size (atrophy) showing consistently 28 % shrinkage of both the right and left cerebral cortex. In most cases, chronic long term dehydration together with chronic acidosis due to poor diet and high cortisol play significant roles in the development of at least three degenerative brain diseases: Stroke, Dementia and Parkinson's.

Stroke

A hemorrhagic stroke is when an artery to the brain tears (dissection) causing bleeding into the brain. This is a very dangerous stroke and frequently results in death. An ischemic stroke, the more common type (85%) of stroke, is when a blood vessel is occluded or blocked (clot) and blood supply and oxygen to the brain is cut off. Stroke is the 3rd leading cause of death in America and it is the leading cause of disability. Strokes affect 15 million Americans and 50% of those over age 85. Those with vascular disease, atherosclerosis or heart disease are at increased risk for stroke. Signs and symptoms of stroke include numbness or weakness on one side of the body - face, arm or leg; loss of speech or vision; confusion; severe headache; loss of balance. Seek medical treatment immediately. Emergency medicine within the first three hours of a stroke can lower glutamate levels in the brain and reduce long term damage and disability.

Causes: Long term use of several prescription medicines which predispose to chronic dehydration and acidosis, poor diet composed primarily of denatured but possibly fortified highly refined processed foods and food substitutes, alcoholism, liver disease, vascular disease, smoking, hypothyroidism, aluminum toxicity from cans (beer and soft drinks) and from cookware, teflon.

Alzheimer's

Alzheimer's is the number one neurological disease in America. It results from the loss of neurons in the highest order areas of the neocortex (new brain), hippocampus (old brain) and amygdala (emotional brain). This manifests as difficulty communicating, getting the right word, memory loss, personality changes, general disorientation and emotional inappropriateness. Alzheimer's has free radical damage in the brain at over twice the rate of patients without dementia, and a loss of up to ten thousand neurons each day. This is associated with disruption of the acetylcholine cycle in the brain (which regulates cognitive function and memory) due to chronic acidosis, malabsorption, malnutrition and dehydration. The Alzheimer's medication Aricept specifically targets increasing the acetylcholine. Only ten percent of Alzheimer's is considered to be due to genetic factors. It is for the most part due to choices of modern life including diet, stress and over medication.

What is loss of cognitive function progressing into dementia like?

A 68 year old man explains to his new girlfriend that things went bad in his last relationship because his girlfriend at the time just stopped making sense. There was lots of anger, he said, and misunderstandings. He has also been very volatile with the new girlfriend, repeatedly calling her crazy and claiming she doesn't make sense and acting out in anger. The first ex-girlfriend was functioning quite well in her very demanding job as a hospital nurse. Only her boyfriend accused her of not making sense, just as he was now saying the same thing about the new girlfriend, though she also was a highly functional medical professional. The gentleman with the cognitive challenge was unable to see the problem as himself, even though the dysfunctional scenarios continued to play out hundreds of times. No amount of explaining to him was having any effect on his outlook as to who wasn't making sense. He was referred for I.V. alpha lipioc acid to improve cognitive function. He indicated on his patient history form that he was unable to get anything done at all - all year, and that he was depressed. Moments later he stated that he did not recognize that he has any psychological or cognitive problems. Pathways in the cerebral cortex necessary to the process of self assessment were damaged.

The sane, healthy, balanced and functional person does not have any power, usually, to get the cognitively impaired individual to recognize which one of them is making sense and which one of them is present to consensus reality - our common shared outlook. It is easy to take the inappropriate behaviors and outlook as a personal affront if one is trying to interact as equals. That is, acting as if both individuals are equally appropriate to time, place and circumstance - each in their own way. Both sides can quickly become defensive and resentful when cognitive impairment is undiagnosed or unacknowledged.

Receiving intravenous ALA for cognitive weakness and brain recovery can produce extreme sleepiness and long periods of deep sleep, as much as 18 to 20 hours. This is because there are a very large percentage of genes for regeneration (about 30%) that are only turned on during sleep and which are turned off while the body is awake. This ALA therapy promotes the body going into that regenerative state that only happens during sleep.

Risk Factors and Causes: Prescription medicines, chronic dehydration due to a diet of highly refined processed foods, chlorine, alcoholism, liver disease, smoking, hypothyroidism, vascular disease, stroke, heart disease, diabetes, and aluminum toxicity possibly from drink cans - beer and sodas (use glass). Alzheimer's brains have been shown to contain up to 30 times more aluminum than normal brains.

The same list of the common risk factors for Alzheimer's are also the risk factors for other degenerative diseases, heart disease, stroke and cancer. Increasing age is a risk factor and half of those over 85 years of age are likely to manifest some degree of Alzheimer's type dementia.

There are also genetic factors affecting lipid and cholesterol functions in the brain. A diet high in unhealthy fats including rancid oils, fried foods and transfats which elevate unhealthy cholesterol and produce obesity will also produce dehydration of the brain and acidosis and sclerosing of normal tissue in the brain, heart and liver. Chronic disorders such as diabetes, hypertension and other sclerosis (harding) of brain tissue (which are often due to life style) are all increased risk factors for dementia. Smoking, alcohol, prescription and non-prescription drugs are all also risk factors for producing Alzheimer's and other dementias.

Diagnosis of mild cognitive impairment is a significant milestone in the development of early stage Alzheimer's. If not effectively reversed at this point there is an 80% to 100% chance of MCI (Mild Cognitive Impairment) progressing to Alzheimer's. Hormone replacement in women over age 65, specifically taking estrogen, is also a factor which increases the risk of dementia and Alzheimer's. Perhaps above all other factors, the persistent chronic stress that causes cortisol flooding and high anxiety actually kills neurons in the brain.

Those common risk factors can mostly be diminished or abated by choosing these ten supportive measures and habits. Eating healthy fats, including omega 3's such as are found in salmon, raw nuts, and oils and supplementing with omegas and CoQ10 are all highly effective in supporting brain health. Maintaining normal weight, avoiding diabetes, obesity and malnutrition are all significant for reducing risk of Alzheimer's and other dementias. Eating healthy fats is the counter point to ending the consumption of unhealthy fats. The brain needs fats but it matters what kind.

Drinking raw juice daily increases nutrition, hydration and pH, all of which are protective of brain health. Including more fresh and particularly raw fruits and vegetables can improve cognitive function. Exercise also improves cognitive function as it stimulates the production of new neurons and essential brain cells.

Continuing the mental, intellectual challenge of learning new skills and active pursuit of personal goals such as writing your book, memories or poetry, composing music, and creating art or crafts all have proven highly effective at reducing the risk of developing Alzheimer's. Laughter, enjoying life, doing what you love and all activities that get more oxytocin flowing including strong social, family and love connections are the best therapy your brain can have. These experiences help us to stay interested and involved in healthy happy ways that produce a strong support system for mental clarity and improved cognitive function. Lowering the stress level by eliminating more of what doesn't work in your life and creating enough down time, balance, sleep and rest is also essential for protecting brain health, memory and cognitive function. Treatment for Alzheimer's tries to replace lost neurons and increase acetylcholine - both of which we can do and perhaps more easily do, with natural therapies to restore normal hydration and optimize pH and nutrition together with a better balance of exercise and stress reduction.

For recovery from Stroke or Alzheimer's consider the use of: Phosphatidyl serine, CoQ10, Floradix liquid vitamins, Vitamin B 100 complex and Folic Acid, alpha lipoic acid, Omega 3 fish oils, Green Vibrance, Penta water (or structured water), Rescue Remedy, Hyperbaric Oxygen, Detoxamin suppositories, I.V. Chelation, raw juice and raw food diet, high protein broth and exercise.

Parkinson's

The second most common neurological disease in America. Presents with signs and symptoms of muscle rigidity, resting tremor, poor balance, lack of muscle control, and involuntary movements. The symptoms are caused by the loss of dopamine in the Central Nervous System due to the death of neurons in the substantia nigra, an area of the mid-brain. Cognition remains normal.

Risk Factors and Causes: exposure to toxic chemicals or heavy metals including Cadmium, petrochemicals (jet fuel), mercury toxicity (use porcelain for dental fillings not amalgam), carbon monoxide poisoning, encephalitis, drugs including prescription drugs, and long term STRESS.

Conventional treatments focus on replacing dopamine which is very difficult because dopamine does not cross the blood brain barrier. Use of Glutathione administered I.V. has been significant, but it can't be taken orally. CoQ10 in very high amounts reduces cortisol binding in the brain and supports oxygenation. Use Penta water, Hyperbaric Oxygen therapy, Floradix liquid vitamins, Vitamin B100 complex, Omegas, Rescue Remedy, no GMO foods.

P.T.S.D.

Post-traumatic stress disorder is a psychiatric diagnosis based on a trauma history which manifests with signs and symptoms of hysteria, loss of control, over reactive due to past trauma, persistent unwanted thoughts, anxiety and/or depression. Also manifests INSOMNIA as a neurohormonal response to severe trauma disrupting the GABA cycle in the brain. Increased and imbalanced levels of epinephrine may also be present. Use 5HTP which is a Serotonin support, structured water, Vitamin B 100 complex, Folic Acid, Floradix, Rescue Remedy, Craniosacral adjustments, Vitamin C for the adrenals, hemp oil, hyperbaric oxygen.

M.S.

Multiple Sclerosis is a central nervous system (CNS) disease which may be chronic or relapsing. It is an autoimmune disease in which the axions of the nerves are demyelinated and can not transmit messages and then these nerves die. Some common signs and symptoms include motor weakness, dropping things, a leg dragging, loss of balance and vision problems.

Risk factors and Causes: Viral infection particularly w/ Echo virus, meningitis or encephalitis, carbon monoxide poisoning, TCE (trichlorethelyne), Celiac disease and candida overgrowth are significant factors and a diet producing chronic acidosis and dehydration speeds deterioration.

Use homeopathy, Structured Water, Hyperbaric Oxygen therapy, Floradix liquid vitamins, Vitamin B100 complex and Folic Acid, flax seed oil, CoQ10, Rescue Remedy, raw juice and raw food diet and exercise.

A.L.S.

Amyotrophic Lateral Sclerosis is a motor neuron disease characterized by a hardening of the lateral portions (sides) of the spine due to astrocyte scarring, an immune system response of the CNS (central nervous system). It presents with gradual progressive loss of voluntary muscle movement and paralysis. Cognition remains intact, but personality changes are likely as disability progresses. Risk factors and Causes: Cadmium, teflon, hypothyroid, chronic stress.

Use Magnesium, Structured water or Penta water, Hyperbaric oxygen treatments, Acetyl L-carnitine, Floradix liquid vitamins, CoQ10, Flax seed oil, Folic Acid, Vitamin B100 complex, Green Vibrance, Rescue Remedy, I.V. DMPS

Treatments:

Super Hydration
Raw juice and raw food to raise pH
High protein broth
Exercise 90 minutes a day 6 days a week
Massage - Reflexology, Craniosacral adjustments
Eat Organic Only. Whole fresh foods, eliminate processed foods, especially grains
Castor oil packs - particularly for Alzheimer's or any liver related cognitive weakness
Kneipp Baths: Hops and Valerian, Lavender
Hyperbaric oxygen

Supplements:

Phospahtidyl Serine - 100 mgs 3 x day for memory and cognitive functions

Alpha Lipoic Acid - 600 mgs 2 x day or intravenous
CoQ10 - 400 to 800 mgs daily, divided dose
Floradix - with Iron and Herbs, Floravital or Epresat
Vitamin B complex - B100's 2 x day
Folic Acid - 800 mcgs daily
Acetyl L-Carnitine - 500 mgs 3 x day, reduces free radical damage
Choline or acetyl choline - neurotransmitter to counter cognitive decline
Coral Calcium - 2,000 mgs per day or Raw Calcium, for dementias involving disruption of the
    calcitonin cycle (hyperthyroid), restlessness, headaches, palpitations and to buffer acidosis
NAC - N -acetyl choline to clear toxins from the brain
5HTP - for Serotonin support
Lithium Orotate - for Serotonin support
Magnesium - for circulation, Floradix liquid or Natural Calm by Natural Vitality
Omegas, fish oils, flax oil and 2 grams 2 x day
DMAE

Hyperbaric Oxygen - pure oxygen under pressure increases O2 saturation and supports cellular
recovery especially for stroke, Parkinson's, MS and brain injury
Structured Water
Rescue Remedy
Detoxamin suppositories for detox - for Alzheimer's and Parkinson's
Green Vibrance for detox, liver and digestive support
Progesterone cream - for women with strokes or any vascular disease, insomnia
Kneipp baths, Valerian and Hops or Lavender for calming. Juniper or Rosemary for stimulating.

Alpha lipoic acid raises glutathione levels and calms excitatory states including elevated glutamate producing seizures. You cannot give the glutathione orally effectively because it doesn't cross the blood brain barrier - but lipoic acid does. I.V. Alpha lipoic acid therapy can in some cases be more effective when preceded by an infusion of I.V. glutathione about one hour before starting the ALA drip.

MOOD ALTERING DRUGS

Hydration, pH and neurochemistry.

In 2005, Americans filled 170 million prescriptions for antidepressants. As a culture, we are addicted to mood altering drugs so that we can continue to do what doesn't work, but feel differently about it. Deficiencies of neurotransmitters (brain chemicals) occur due to nutritional deficiencies, chronic dehydration, acidosis, increased toxic burden and traumas. The result is depression, anxiety, OCD, (attention deficit disorder,) and many other states of cognitive and emotional impairment. The limbic system of the brain has functions for pleasure, happiness, joy, mood fluctuations, personality and temperament, memory, emotional learning, sleep, arousal and alertness. It is a neurological feedback loop which regulates mood and compares it to past experience. Personality and morality have specific locations in the brain and any disruption of the balance of excitatory and inhibitory neurotransmitters produces changes in the psychological state and can manifest as mental emotional illness.

The two most common sources of brain chemistry imbalance today are the acid forming diet of refined processed foods which results in demineralization for acid buffering and, similarly, the cumulative effect of multiple prescription medications, particularly when continued for a period of many years. Both of these challenges also produce chronic subclinical dehydration further contributing to the disruption of the acetyl choline cycle of the brain. This reduces mental clarity, inhibits cognitive function and impairs memory, each of which contributes to frustration, irritation and stress. Long term continuous use of prescription sleep aids and anti-depressants impair brain health through diminished cerebral circulation, reduction of nutrient transfer and waste elimination in brain tissue and widespread sclerosing (hardening) of the brain tissue.

Treatment to reverse the damage caused by dehydration and acidosis in the brain includes a therapeutic diet of whole, fresh, unprocessed foods with an emphasis on 50% or more raw food to raise pH as quickly as possible and to increase hydration which in turn provides support for more efficient kidney and liver functions to help restore normal brain chemistry.

Neuronutrients to support healthy brain tissue and supplements to promote detoxing of brain tissue may be needed until both mood and brain health improve. Remember, you can't just stop taking medications. You have to make the necessary changes and do what it takes to heal and not need the medications so enlist the support of your doctor in discontinuing prescriptions you may no longer need.

Nutritional deficiencies greatly contribute to brain and mind/emotion imbalances. These can develop through: Leaky Gut Syndrome, antibiotic therapy, yeast overgrowth called Candida, Celiac or gluten sensitivity, parasites, iron deficiency, iodine, calcium and magnesium deficiencies and deficiency of the agent of calcium transport, (vitamin D used up in a process of demineralization to buffer acidoses).

Treatments:

Therapeutic doses of acidophilus 3 times a day, Floradix with iron & herbs, quercetin for allergic reactions, greens to support healthy blood, liver health and detoxing, structured water to reverse dehydration, raw juice, high protein broth.

Hormone imbalance - Low progesterone and progesterone precursor pregnenalone, thyroid imbalance, and adrenal cortisol flooding can exist separately or simultaneously and all have profound effects on mood and personality. Steroids lower CoQ10 by 50% because the body uses up all the CoQ10 available to stop cortisol binding to neurons.

Heavy metals and toxins cause depression and anxiety: mercury, cadmium, lead, arsenic, pesticide, fertilizers, chlorine, PCB's.
Treatment - colonics, Detoxamin suppositories and Calcium Disodium EDTA either orally or by I.V. infusion.

Trauma - emotional and physical. Treatment - process work and cognitive behavior therapy, EFT, talk therapy and group therapy and counseling of all kinds, hypnosis.

Supplying the essential amino acid precursors and cofactors together with a diet of whole, fresh food, adequate hydration with pure water and sufficient exercise to build strength and stamina is the best support system for healing mood disorders due to imbalances of neurochemistry.

Dopamine Cycle	Amino Acid Precursor	Drugs
attention, focus, pleasure addictions of every kind	Tyrosine, phenylalanine, disrupted by lead, chlorine and history of addiction	Wellbutrin, Ritalin

Serotonin Cycle		
joy, sleep, irritability, libido, OCD, Panic, PMS	Tryptophan, 5HTP, DHA, DMAE disrupted by trauma, arsenic, mercury, extreme stress or hysteria	Prozac, Lexapro, Zoloft

Increasing levels increases sense of well being disrupted by history of drug addiction.

Acetylcholine Cycle	
cognitive functions, memory, dementia	Choline, phospyhtidyl serine, acetyl L-carnitine, Floradix, Folic acid, B-complex, SAM-e, calcium, copper, progesterone, quercitin, disrupted by acidosis, steroids, antidepressants or Ambien, adrenal exhaustion, malnutrition, chemicals

Gaba Cycle

| panic / anxiety limbic system | Exercise, CoQ10, Omegas, Lithium orotate, I.V. glutathione disrupted by dehydration, trauma | Xanex, Klonapin, Ambien |

GABA is the main inhibitory or calming neurotransmitter.

Oxytocin - social bonding, sexual bonding. The love molecule. Drug: Ecstasy

Opioids - endorphins regulate the transmission of emotional and physical pain.

Norepinephrine - sleep wake cycle, attention, blood flow to brain, sense of well being.

Glutamate - main excitatory neurotransmitter in Central Nervous System. Can cause seizures, hyperactivity disorders.

An average urine pH below 6 is too acidic. Ideal is 6.5 to 7. A urine pH below 5.4 is a state of acidosis which will produce biochemical anomalies throughout the body, including disturbances in the acetylcholine cycle in the brain. This is a factor in cognitive decline and dementia. Dehydration also disrupts the GABA cycle in the brain, producing panic attacks and chronic anxiety. Prescriptions for mood altering drugs further contribute to dehydration and to the toxic burden, which further acidifies the body.

Mood Altering Drugs: You can physically alter your mood by inhaling doTERRA, Certified Pure Therapeutic Grade essential oils. Elevation and Frankincense to feel inspired and encourged, Citrus Bliss to feel motivated and uplifted, Serenity to feel calm and peaceful, Balance to feel grounded and reassured.

The physiologic reward system is activated by food, drink, sex, drugs and pleasure of all kinds, but especially by the anticipation of pleasure under conditions of uncertainty as to obtaining it. Oxytocin, dopamine and endorphins are all reward system neurotransmitters. An imbalance in any of them can produce the experience of depression. The human brain is hardwired to seek happiness and joy because it is beneficial for health; and because it is a profoundly effective guidance towards the fulfillment of the soul's purpose for incarnating.

> **"The soul is happy by nature; the soul is happiness itself. It becomes unhappy when something is the matter with its vehicle, its instrument, its tool through which it experiences life. Care of the body, therefore, is the first and most important principal of religion."**
>
> **Inayat Khan**

Migraine / Headaches

General picture - usually an escalating toxic reading together with dehydration (often -3 or below, but not always) and overwhelming stress of +5 to +8, always. About 75% of migraines involve adrenal exhaustion. Excessive blood flow congested to the brain with vascular tension triggered by dehydration due to toxic overload is occurring in about 60% of migraines, and may cause nausea and vomiting. Migraines are a central nervous system disorder and are the result of a disruption in the serotonin dopamine balance 15% of the time, disruption of acetylcholine cycle 60% of the time and inhibited norepinephrine 92% of the time.

Treatments:

Super Hydrate - with 4 liters of Penta or more and Bach Flower: Sweet Chestnut
Reflexology - hands and feet to balance circulation, lymphatic drainage
Enemas or Basti - 12 oz. water with 3 oz. oil (flax or castor) every 10 days x 4 repetitions
Elimination Diet. Avoid MSG - often in broth. Avoid chocolate, corn syrup, oranges and alcohol.
Fasting and modified fasting provide relief.
Soak feet in hot water
Kneipp Hops and Valerian bath
Exercise 60 minutes a day 6 days a week
Brain levels of glutamate - the excitatory neurotransmitter will be elevated.
Use alpha lipoic acid to raise glutathione and balance glutamate.
Hyperbaric Oxygen

Supplements & Botanicals:

Acidophilus - mixed or Reuteri
Fresh ginger tea - 4 to 6 cups daily
5 HTP - 300 mgs 2 x day - tryptophan
CoQ10 - 400 mgs 2 x day
Folic Acid - 800 mcgs
Evening Primrose Oil - 2,000 mgs 2 x day or Omegas
Pycnogenols - 300 mgs 2 x day
Digestive Enzymes - 3 x day
Thyrocalm by Wilson's - for hormone balance
Heavy Metal detox - Mercury and Fluoride (calcium disodium EDTA)
Rescue Remedy

To heal the underlying factors predisposing to migraine, it is necessary to heal the adrenals in order to balance the brain chemistry. This means healing patterns which promote chronic stress, healing trauma and finding and maintaining sustainable balance between levels of activity and repose.

VISION HEALTH

Eyes age along with the rest of the body. Vision weakens when chronic high blood sugar damages blood vessels, toxic build up damages lenses and build up of pressure damages the optic nerve and retina. Protecting vision health is directly related to maintaining overall general health through diet, exercise and stress reduction. Eye strain is a form of physical stress indicating that visual acuity is diminishing at the level of the brain. The eyes, or rather the optic nerve specifically, is brain tissue. The rods (light sensitive) and cones (color sensitive) of the eye are receptor cells sending electrochemical signals to the brain from which the brain constructs the visual image. Brain health is essential to vision health. The eyes transmit about one billion bits of information to the brain per second. From this, the brain chooses selective visual awareness.

One common type of vision impairment occurs because the retina becomes less sensitive to light and thus brighter light is required to see well. Equally common is the sclerosing or hardening of the lens which reduces its ability to change shape in order to adjust focus. Evidence of this type of lens hardening is loss of ability to see small writing and to see at very close range. High blood pressure and diabetes also contribute to blurring of vision.

Many prescription and over the counter drugs also cause damage to the optic nerve, retina and optic vessels. Medications for gout and diabetes, steroids, aspirin, diuretics, antihistamines, psychotropic drugs, quinine, and anti-coagulants are just some of the many common drugs that are known to have detrimental effects on vision health. In addition to the damage done by the medication, the underlying condition for which it is being used is probably also causing a significant loss of visual health.

The health of the eyes, as to dry, watery, burning, irritated, itchy, over sensitive to light, swollen lids and dark circles, all serve as windows to a deeper disturbance such as allergies, liver disease, high blood pressure and adrenal exhaustion. Vision weakens with most major health challenges including cancer, heart disease and diabetes because all of these are states of biochemical imbalance that directly damage the delicate tissues of the eye, including its circulatory vessels, its lens, retina and associated nerves. Leaky vessels of the neural retina reflect a similar weakness in the vessels of the brain.

Supplements specifically for support of vision health include lutein, vitamin C, vitamin B, essential fatty acids called omegas and vitamin A.

Lutein is a carotenoid, meaning it is of the vitamin A family. Lutein is particularly concentrated in the tissues of the eye lens and macular pigment. Food sourced and dietary concentration of lutein from spinach and egg yolks are particularly significant for minimizing retinal degeneration and inhibiting cataract development. Lutein protects the macula from oxidative stress.

Cataracts

A cataract is a cloudy lens. This clouding of the lens is due to biochemical changes in the lens itself. Surgery replaces the damaged lens with an artificial lens. This age related accumulation of opaque proteins on the lens is experienced by well more than 50% of those past age 70. For those at highest risk, smokers and diabetics, the cataracts may develop by age 60. Frequent exposure to intense direct sunlight without the protection of sunglasses also contributes significantly to acceleration of the formation of cataracts.

Macular Degeneration

This degeneration of the central vision is a leading cause of blindness in the elderly. The macula is a central area of the retina. The deterioration of the rods, cones and cells of this area (at the center back of the eye) causes visual distortion, blurring and eventually a blank spot in the visual field. The cells that are degrading are normally particularly rich in the carotenoid lutein which has been shown to slow this process of cell destruction. The leaky vessels in the eye are usually a reflection of poor circulatory health. Atherosclerosis, diabetes and smoking are all high risk factors for this type of vision loss. A diet of unhealthy saturated fats, trans fats and rancid oils rapidly increases the rate of cell destruction and loss of vision.

Glaucoma

Glaucoma is a disease of increased pressure within the eye which is also a leading cause of blindness. This build up of pressure is due to a sclerosing and clogging of tissue that functions to drain fluid from the eye. Chronic dehydration, alcohol and smoking all damage this delicate sponge-like tissue and inhibit its function of supplying nutrients and removing wastes from the eye. Diabetes and high blood sugar, chronic high stress and medications (including antihistamines, steroids and blood pressure drugs) are all known to increase pressure in the eyes which destroys peripheral vision. Omega fatty acids are the supplement most supportive to healing glaucoma.

Conjunctivitis

Inflammation of the membranes of the eye can be caused by bacterial or viral infection and by allergic reaction to irritants such as smoke. Redness, tears, mucus discharge and sensitivity to light usually last several days and then clear up. Some forms of conjunctivitis are highly contagious and most often a trip to the doctor for speedy relief is well indicated. Conjunctivitis happens at any age: infants, children, adults and elderly.

EARS AND HEARING HEALTH

Hearing Loss

Hearing loss can begin at any age. If it has existed since birth, hearing loss may not improve at all with natural healing methods. If the onset of hearing loss is due to injury or illness causing structural or tissue damage, including mild scarring, it is probably at least partially reversible over time by optimizing circulatory health and overall general health. Food allergies to grains are a factor in 45% of cases and medication is a factor in 30% of cases. Radiation treatment for brain cancer also produces deafness about 40% of the time. The number one cause of hearing loss is the sclerosing of the three tiny bones of the middle ear. Damage to the cilia (hairs) of the cochlea and damage to the auditory nerve are the other leading causes. The facial nerve for the stapedius muscle and the trigeminal nerve for the tensor tympani muscle may also be involved.

Dizzy Spells

Vertigo, nausea and a sensation of spinning are all caused by a disturbance of the inner ear. In some cases, this is a problem of calcium crystals in the fluid of the cochlea. This can produce disorientation and may precede a stroke.

Tinnitus

Hearing continuous or intermittent ringing in the ears is called tinnitus. It is a stimulation of the auditory nerve that is produced through elevated blood pressure in cerebral circulation. The three main causal factors are dehydration, stress, and elevated blood pressure. Learning conscious relaxation to lower stress levels together with improving hydration and pH to take the burden off the kidneys and improve blood pressure will resolve most tinnitus in 60 to 90 days. However, poor cerebral circulation, high blood pressure and acidosis causes a hardening of the tiny bones of the inner ear called otosclerosis. This condition often accompanies osteoporosis, advancing Alzheimer's and stroke. If the tinnitus has persisted for over two years and otosclerosis has developed, the tinnitus may become irreversible. Certain medications, including antibiotics and quinine are also promoters of tinnitus. Cranio sacral adjustments are recommended. Aromatherapy: doTerra Helichrysum. Use hemp oil to lower cortisol levels.

Intense exposure to sound, jack hammers and rock bands causes damage to the tiny hairs that pick up the audio vibrations from the fluid in the cochlea. Though this is often suggested as a cause for tinnitus, in the readings it corresponds to hearing loss and not to tinnitus. This kind of hearing loss is not reversible and may require an assisted listening device. The hearing aid will not improve the tinnitus, but it also will not amplify or aggravate it.

Ear Infections

May include congestion and infection, ear ache, usually pain, pressure and fever. Outer ear infection is on the external side of the ear drum and can be caused by water that remains in the ear. A deeper infection, otitis media, is usually due to the build up of mucus and pressure in the inner ear related to congestion, coughing and nose blowing. These ear infections are bacterial and usually respond well to antibiotics. Sometimes antibiotics can be avoided by the use of well indicated homeopathic remedies such as Nat. Mur. or Pulsatilla. Ear infections are often related to food allergies and sinus infections. Aromatherapy: doTerra Helichrysum.

Ear Candles - not really a candle at all but about the size and shape of an ordinary taper, the ear candle is really an open tube. With a flame lighted at its outer point, the ear candle creates a gentle vacuum that pulls wax and debris out of the ear canal. Each ear candle takes 15 to 20 minutes to burn down and each ear may require two candles to remove the obstructions and clear the channel to improve hearing. This is not a treatment for ear infection. It is an effective treatment for impacted wax. It also has benefits similar to cranial adjustment. The use of an open flame requires specific precautions including a bowl of water for dousing flames instantly when required.

Hearing Voices

The phenomena of clairaudience is perhaps distinguishable from mental illness only in the quality of the audio content. If the voices in your head offer consistently beneficial guidance, then it is considered clairaudience. If one hears voices, or anything else that others don't hear, and it causes inappropriate behaviors in response, then it qualifies as mental illness.

My experience of clairaudience is that it is an experience of inner hearing that takes place through perception of subtle vibrations moving in the fluid of the cochlea. It is not a sound outside the self that is perceived through highly developed senses, but rather it is a sound that emerges from within, from the soul's knowing. Some moments of clairaudience seem intensely 'out loud' as they resonate in one's being. Other times the hearing is a more subtle experience. To cultivate clairaudience, spend many hours a day in silence. Be still and know.

CIRCULATORY HEALTH

Circulatory health is essential to the overall life of the human organism and to each and every cell as well. The adult body has 60,000 miles of blood vessels. The durability and tension in the vein walls, the unobstructed passibility of blood vessels, the vigor of the heart pumping the blood and the blood chemistry itself (including glucose, calcium, copper, magnesium, potassium, salt, iron and oxygen as well as clotting factors) are all significant factors which together determine circulatory health. In addition, there are significant subcategories of circulation with specific therapeutic implications including cerebral circulation (brain), coronary circulation (heart), hepatic circulation (liver) and systemic circulation. Circulatory health covers a wide range of disease manifestations including angina, anemia, arrhythmia, congestive heart failure, high blood pressure, varicose veins, aneurism and stroke, atherosclerosis, and heart attack. Circulatory failure of some form is the most frequent cause of death and heart attack is the most frequent of all. Risk factors for circulatory health include diabetes, smoking, high blood pressure, birth control pills, alcohol, malnutrition, dehydration and chronic high stress.

Angina

Angina is a pain in the chest which may radiate to the left arm, neck, face or back. Functionally, it is like a heart attack but milder. It is a serious warning from the body and warrants a medical check up by your doctor. Angina can be triggered by emotional stress, extreme exertion, alcohol, cigarettes and also at night during sleep when blood pressure drops.

Arrhythmia

Arrhythmia means irregular heart beat. If natural therapies (including diet, hydration, supplements and stress management) fail to regulate the heart beat within three weeks, seek the guidance of a trained professional. Yoga and conscious relaxation may be particularly effective at stabilizing heart rhythms.

Congestive Heart Failure

Congestive heart failure, also called cardiac insufficiency, means a loss of vigor due to a weakened, damaged, exhausted heart which is incapable of pumping blood adequately, resulting in swollen feet, legs and ankles, fatigue and respiratory distress.

Atherosclerosis

Atherosclerosis, the most common circulatory disease, is a sclerosing or hardening and an unhealthy build up of cells on blood vessel walls. Also called coronary artery disease, this circulatory weakness affects 60 million Americans. This hardening and blockage of blood vessels is due to unhealthy blood chemistry producing an oxidation of cholesterol. Cholesterol is necessary for health, but abnormal blood chemistry factors including high cortisol, acid pH and dehydration together with chemical environmental toxins all cause healthy cholesterol to oxidize into unhealthy cholesterol. Atherosclerosis produces heart attacks which are episodes of interruption of blood supply to the heart. If a heart attack is survived, it can produce lasting damage resulting in cardiac insufficiency and degenerative heart disease.

High Blood Pressure

High blood pressure is also a circulatory weakness or disease that is causally related to heart disease, stress management and exercise as well as pH (because it affects kidney function), and hydration. Medications used to lower blood pressure are designed to produce the same effect in the body that increased water intake would produce. Why not just prescribe water and responsible hydration, instead of pills? Some patients will not comply with sustainable hydration but are more likely to rely on the convenience of pills to control their problem. This means not solving for the problem itself and restoring health, and therefore, results only in symptomatic control while the underlying causal factors remain unaddressed and the overall general health deteriorates.

Patients are often able to get off of blood pressure medication just by consuming a lot more raw fruits and vegetables which raises potassium levels, enzyme levels, pH and hydration. Omega 3 fatty acids also support healthy blood pressure and improved circulation by opening vessels and healing the walls of the blood vessels. CoQ10 supports both heart health and blood vessel health and significantly improves oxygenation and vitality. Supplemental calcium has been shown to lower serum cholesterol and is also a factor in circulatory health. Vasoconstriction is also triggered by magnesium depletion. Vasoconstriction produces heart attacks as well as the peripheral circulatory insufficiency that is produced with diabetes (wherein capillary circulation fails due to high blood glucose and dehydration). This results in poor wound healing and amputation of limbs.

For serious circulatory problems including coronary artery disease and heart attack recovery and prevention, chelation with intravenous EDTA is frequently recommended. EDTA chelation therapy is an amino acid-like molecule that binds with metals and toxins in the blood and promotes more effective excretion of these oxidizing elements from the body.

Anemia

Anemia is a weakness of the chemical composition of the blood. The most common type of anemia is iron deficiency anemia but there are many others. Anemia produces generalized weakness and loss of vitality, exhaustion, fainting and dizzy spells.

Varicose Veins

Varicose veins are another common circulatory weakness. Varicose veins are visible through the skin and may be swollen, even lumpy. Weakness of the blood vessel walls which produce varicosities are due to consumption of unhealthy fats together with high blood glucose levels due to sugar and starch and may be greatly predisposed by heredity.

Treatments:

For effective treatment of circulatory weakness, consider all of the following factors: Emotions, hydration, blood thinners including vitamin C, vitamin E, progesterone and aspirin; minerals including potassium, magnesium, copper, iron; healthy fats including alpha lipoic acid and omega 3 fatty acids; CoQ10; the B vitamin, niacin, which dilates blood vessels somewhat like nitroglycerin does; and the botanicals hawthorne berry, Ginko and ginger. For body mind support consider yoga, journaling, music to lower stress, massage and aromatherapy. In all cases, exercise to increase stamina, flexibility and resilience is absolutely essential to recovery of circulatory health.

Hypertension

High Blood Pressure is 140 to 160 over 100
Stage 3 hypertension is 180 to 200 over 110 to 120
About 30% of Americans over age 30 will experience bouts of high blood pressure. Sometimes there are no obvious symptoms. It can cause headaches, nosebleeds, palpitations, tension, anxiety, and ringing in the ears. The heart is working harder, predisposing to a heart attack, stroke and kidney failure.

All common BP meds are known to cause impotence and decreased libido including ace inhibitors, vasodilators and beta blockers. Ace inhibitors are also associated with persistent cough as a side effect.

Spiritual:

Repressed emotions, FEAR, trauma.

Causes:

Chronic dehydration due to toxic overload including caffeine, alcohol and drugs, including steroids, prescription and over the counter medications, recreational drugs, chocolate, a typical American diet of highly processed refined foods and 20% or more of calories from sugar. OBESITY - Blood Pressure drops with weight loss. Diabetes, kidney disease, adrenal disorder - cortisol function/fight or flight response to chronic stress, worry, anxiety, family conflicts, hostility, anger, smoking and chewing tobacco. Nicotine is vasoconstrictive. Pregnancy (due to increased blood volume or toxemia), physical inactivity, tumor.

Treatments:

Lifestyle moderation
Hydration -12 glasses of structured water daily with fresh lemon
Elimination Diet - EAT WHOLE FRESH FOODS
Breathing Exercises. Meditation. Relaxation training. Music.
Aromatherapy. Kneipp Valerian and Hops Bath
Exercise - Tai Chi, Yoga, Walking, 45 to 60 minutes 6 days a week (or 7)
Bodywork - Reflexology, Craniaosacral adjustment, neuro-muscular massage and Acupuncture

Supplements:

Nordic Naturals ProOmega fish oils 1,000 mgs caps - 2 caps 2 x day
CoQ10 - 300 to 400 mgs 2 x day
Magnesium gluconate - 500 mgs 2 x day
Potassium - 2000 mgs 2 x day (fruits and vegetables)
Phosphytidyl Serine - 200 mgs 2 x day
Vitamin E - 800 I.U.'s daily, use pure d-alpha tocopherol (not mixed tocopherols)
Wilson's HTN
Hawthorne berry - 500 mgs in the morning, vasodilator

Maitaike mushrooms
Foods - spinach, asparagus, bananas, apricots, dates, raisins, prunes, watermelon, pomegranate, raw juice and increase raw food

Heart Disease

Affects 60 million Americans. Atherosclerosis is the leading cause of disability and death. 1 in 4 Americans dies of heart disease. Heart attacks were rare before the 1920's when manufactured cigarettes became available and highly processed refined flour products.

Causes:

Caused by poor dietary choices, chronic STRESS and regular use of coffee and alcohol, 20% of calories from sugar. Lack of exercise. Predisposing factors include obesity, smoking, diabetes, high blood pressure, high cholesterol, genetics, sedentary lifestyle, lack of physical fitness, low testosterone. Heart disease is reversible. It causes fatigue, shortness of breath and swollen ankles.

Emotions:

Anxiety, unloved, unloveable

Treatment:

Stop Smoking
Diet - whole, fresh, unprocessed foods. Decrease saturated fats.
Structured water - 2.5 to 3 liters daily
Chelation with EDTA or DMPS
DETOXIFICATION with greens, bitters, enemas, Flor-Essence. Aromatherapy - Lavender
RELAXATION, Meditation, Stress Management, Forgiveness, Trust.
Breathing Exercises
Bodywork - Neuromuscular massage, Rolfing
EXERCISE lowers risk of heart attack by 50%

Supplements:

B vitamins - 800 mcgs of Folic Acid and vitamin B 100 complex, once or twice a day
CoQ10 - 300 to 400 mgs 2 x day

Vitamin E - 800 I.U.'s per day
Magnesium gluconate - 500 mgs 2 x day
Fish Oils - Nordic Naturals Complete Omega 1,000 mgs caps - 2 or 3 caps 2 times a day
Selenium - for arrythmias - 850 mcgs per day
L-Carnitine - 3 grams per day
Testosterone for men, requires medical supervision
Hawthorne berry capsules - 500 mgs, vasodilator once or twice a day
Watermelon seed tea - diuretic
Fresh ginger tea - 5 cups per day

Healing heart disease means having a change of heart about day to day choices, personality, diet, exercise and spiritual practice. Discovery of how to create happiness in one's daily life is fundamental to heart health.

RESPIRATORY HEALTH

The group of illnesses called respiratory disease are among the most common in America and world wide. This is because the lungs filter our air which is increasingly laden with toxic pollution as well as viruses, mold, bacteria and other particulate matter. About a third of Americans experience respiratory challenges regularly as colds, sinus infections, hay fever and bronchitis as well as the more serious diseases asthma, pneumonia and emphysema.

Ear infections are considered a form of respiratory infection because they most often originate from the same infections that are producing colds, flu and sinus infection. Chronic sinusitis and allergies are usually manifested under high stress physically and psychologically together with the burden of a toxic diet and toxic air supply, perhaps both indoors and outside. Wheat and all processed grains are the most common cause of respiratory symptoms we call allergies, even though the offending agent is a food allergen. Dairy, especially industrial grade dairy with its heavy chemical burden of antibiotics, hormones, fertilizers and herbicides (glyphosate) is the second most common cause of sinus infection. Reactions to these foods also contributes to the growth of nasal polyps and enlarged adenoids.

Most people who seek symptomatic relief from chronic sinusitis or hay fever never choose to do anything to overcome the underlying problems. We take the convenient way of believing these things just happen, through no specific action on our part but the truth is, nothing is without cause. Overall general health including the resilience of being well rested, the vigor of physical fitness and strength of psychological balance and inner peace is all manifesting some effect in the breath and plays a role in respiratory health.

Unhappiness in the form of deep grief is particularly associated with the lungs and with respiratory health. Fear and trust issues are also prominent in chronic respiratory weakness. Meditation, journaling and emotional release work are all highly effective tools for improving respiratory health. Weight and exercise also regulate respiratory health. Exercise develops the depth and rhythm of the breath. Lighter weight and flat belly reduce the burden on respiratory functions whereas the excess weight and abdominal constrictions and pressure on the diaphragm make it much more difficult to breathe, particularly right after eating.

Asthma

Reactive airway syndrome. Characterized by episodes of respiratory distress in response to various triggers including emotional, physical stress, over heating, exercise induced asthma, pollen, dander, smoke, chemicals - especially cleaning agents, over eating, food allergies and other acute respiratory illness such as colds, bronchitis, flu and pneumonia. Acute shortness of breath, gasping, wheezing and coughing are the symptoms of asthma attack. Occasionally, gagging or fainting may also occur.
Asthma is a combination of unresolved trauma and anxiety together with a frailty of constitution and overall general health. During an asthma attack, bronchioles constrict and mucus production increases and exchange of oxygen is reduced.

Asthma is a chronic deteriorating disease that can be quite debilitating (except when it isn't). Learning to manage asthma when acute episodes occur is of vital importance. Often an inhaler is required, and the bronchodilator albuterol is one of the most effective inhaler dispensed asthma medications available.

Bronchitis

Inflammation of the membrane lining the bronchial tubes which causes congestion, swollen tissues, cough and impaired respiration, short winded. Usually there is fever and generalized illness as well.

Steam humidifiers, vaporizers and steamy showers provide temporary relief. Avoiding dairy and grains, unhealthy fats and processed foods generally reduces congestion and slows mucus production. Fasting and modified fasting on broth, speed recovery time.

Hot teas and hot lemon honey water help relax the chest muscles and constricted air ways while supporting hydration which always falls during any acute illness. Oral vitamin C several times a day and oregano oil capsules provide extra support for recovery.

Pneumonia

A more serious infection than bronchitis, pneumonia can be caused by bacterial infection, virus, fungal infection or mold and chemical exposures. This is a common illness, in one of these forms, and usually manifests significant fever, pain in the chest or back and cough. Oxygen efficiency diminishes rapidly as lung tissue fills with fluid and breathing becomes labored. Fasting on broth, raw juice or structured water can greatly speed recovery while over eating and poor food choices can delay recovery.

The acute symptoms of pneumonia can linger for weeks, and full recovery often takes months with high incidence of relapse. When ability to recover is poor, consider intravenous Vitamin C to provide quick relief and shorten the overall duration of illness. Aromatherapy: doTerra Oregano oil (also internally).

Emphysema

Emphysema and chronic bronchitis, which together are also called COPD or chronic obstructive pulmonary disease, are caused primarily by cigarettes or other directly inhaled toxins. This is degenerative lung disease characterized by moderate to severe shortness of breath and susceptibility to repeated acute respiratory infections that can rapidly develop into fatal pneumonia. Lung function is gradually lost due to hardening and scarring of lung tissue which can then no longer exchange lung gases normally. Supplemental oxygen therapy becomes increasingly necessary. Vitamin C, CoQ10, Omega 3's and vitamin A are also needed. Digestive enzymes are recommended with every meal and snack.

Respiratory

Asthma, Pneumonia, Emphysema
Chronic lung disease is the 4th leading cause of death in the United States.
Tightness of chest, difficulty breathing, wheezing, cough, reactions to pollen, dander, smoke, mold, air pollution, chemicals and stress.

Emotions:

Trust issues, feelings of inadequacy, grief

Treatments:

Breathing Exercises. Meditation, mindful breathing. Steam inhalation. Eliminate Smoking.
Exercise 60 minutes per day
Lose weight
Enemas to relieve toxic burden (or Dr. Miller's Holy Tea) Castor oil packs over abdomen/omentum.
HYDRATION - 12 cups of water daily. add Rescue Remedy for extra support.
Aromatherapy diffuser: doTerra OnGuard, Eucalyptus or Peppermint. (OnGuard is doTerra's version of the ancient Thieves blend), Thieves by Young Living, (which is clove, cinnamon, lemon, eucalyptus, rosemary).

Kneipp Baths - Eucalyptus.

Supplements:

Probiotics for upper and lower digestive Sambuguard - Elderbery, echinacea and vitamin C
CoQ10 - 300 to 400 mgs 2 x day
Green Vibrance - (probiotics and greens)
Quercetin - up to 4 grams per hour x 3 hours, then 3 to 4 grams 3 x day (antihistamine)
Vitamin B 100 Complex - 2 x day
GSE - grapefruit seed extract, 3 drops in water 3 x a day.
Antimicrobial, antiviral. Shiitaki mushrooms
Cayenne pepper
Vitamin C - 3 grams per dose 3 x day x 8 weeks, then reduce

Diet:

Modified fasting to cleanse toxic overload, raw juice, broth, digestive enzymes, acidophilus - full spectrum.
Elimination diet - chocolate, alcohol, grains, dairy, citrus, pesticides.
Blood Type Diet
Hot drinks - cinnamon stick tea, fresh ginger tea
Eat small meals of easily digestible fresh foods, soups and broths.

Bodywork:

Osteopathic adjustment, deep tissue massage

Allergies, Sinus Infection

INTOLERANCE
Allergy is an immune response. Seventy percent of the immune system is in the gut and thus the digestive system is often the underlying weakness behind allergies and 85% of sinus infections. The usual cause is chronic dehydration due to highly processed refined foods, especially wheat, soy, corn syrup, alcohol, chocolate and coffee. Dehydration also results from use of prescription and over the counter sinus and allergy medicines, pain relievers, anti-anxiety and antidepressants, sleep aids and many others. Leaky Gut syndrome is behind 70% of allergies and 55% of sinus infections. Healing the gut heals the sinuses and nasal passages as well as the respiratory system

which is on the same meridian as the large intestine. Cracks inside the nose correspond to inflammation in the descending colon.

Causes:

dehydration, diet, air pollution, smoke, toxic fumes, mold, antibiotics and yeast overgrowth, stress and persistent anger. Types - seasonal and pollen related, food related, environmental and stress/anger related

Symptoms:

Head congestion, facial pain, fatigue (adrenal exhaustion), sneezing, itching, coughing, wheezing and rashes

Treatments:

Elimination Diet. Eat whole, fresh, organic only for 6 months. Modified fasting.
Colonics every 14 days for 3 repetitions
Edgar Cayce Castor Oil packs over abdomen and descending colon every 3 days for 20 repetitions of 3 hours each
Massage - lymphatic drainage
Adrenal support - physical fitness

Supplements And Botanicals:

Increase structured water to 12 cups daily or use Penta water
Probiotics - mixed.
Green Vibrance Digestive Enzymes 3x day
Fresh ginger tea - 5 cups daily. No sugar, use Agave sweetener
Quercetin - 3 grams 2 or 3 x a day - (instead of Claritin or Zyrtec), inhibits auto immune response and allergic symptoms
Vitamin C 3x day x 3 grams per dose for 2 weeks then reduce to 2 grams per dose
    Vitamin C is the frequency of kindness and supports adrenal recovery from stress
SambuGuard - Elderberry syrup, echinacea & vitamin C, supports the immune system
GSE - grapefruit seed extract, 4 x per day, 3 drops in water or 2 capsules per dose
Colostrum
Dr. Miller's Holy Tea - to cleanse and heal the intestines, supports detoxing
Raw greens, supports detox and cleanses colon. Eat 30% to 40% raw diet.

Avoid grains. Most sinus allergies are from the gut and are caused or aggravated especially by processed grains - wheat, corn, soy - as well as over consumption of processed foods in general. Bach Rescue Remedy drops and pastilles for acute attack

Life Threatening Allergies

Life threatening allergies are significantly different than seasonal allergies such as "hay fever". An anaphylactic emergency may begin with respiratory distress, swelling lips and hives and progresses rapidly into panic, shock and death from respiratory and circulatory failure. Treatment for anaphylaxis is always epinephrine, which can be administered with an injection by an EpiPen, and an emergency call to 911 to stabilize and transport the patient to the hospital.

This life threatening allergic response can be triggered by foods (including peanuts and tree nuts), insect bites or stings (bees), medicines and latex in those individuals who are susceptible. Vulnerability to this potentially fatal allergic reaction may be completely unknown until the onset of the first anaphylactic episode. Once this dangerous sensitivity to allergic reactions has been identified, the individual (or caregivers) can be prescribed an EpiPen and trained in how to use it for immediate emergency support. The website allergyhome.org can be a valuable source of information for those families learning to manage the challenges of life threatening allergies.

The Joys of Raising Our Severely Allergic Child
by Annette Crotti

This is a story about our precious daughter, Alexandra, and the journey we have encountered in managing her allergies and immune challenges.

She was born in 1998 and experienced digestive challenges immediately after birth. Attempts to modify my diet, as a nursing mother, did not make a significant impact. Sadly, I experienced milk production problems, and Alexandra was prematurely weaned at three months. Through trial and error, including the severest response from a soy formula (requiring her to be treated as a burn victim with Dromeboro soaks) we wound up with a predigested formula that she survived on for two years. Even so, she was allergic to the corn syrup it contained; and therefore endured a rash most days. Within that period of time, we cautiously experimented with foods and worked to build up her immune system with probiotics and homeopathic remedies. Eventually, she was able to tolerate a very strict vegetarian rotation diet. A high emphasis was placed on soups and food that was easily digestible, so as not to over tax her system, allowing for maturity.

Our choice to manage Alexandra's allergies in this manner was based on our previous experience with chronic, unexplainable allergies of her mother, (myself). After decades of dead ends resulting in over use of steroids and antihistamines only to experience a worsening of symptoms, I chose to explore alternatives that would eventually lead to my relationship with Fravarti. Prior to learning about Classical Homeopathy, I experimented with other modalities, many of which alleviated symptoms temporarily and taught me to make different lifestyle choices.

Once I began constitutional work with Kentian style homeopathy, I was able to enjoy improved health. It became apparent that there are alternatives to drugs that would eventually harm organs and systems, although the cost would be lifestyle choices that might go against conventional wisdom and our culture at large. Most are unwilling to practice complete avoidance of possible allergens, food as medicine (including daily smoothies or extraction juice), probiotic and digestive enzyme support along with other supplements, attention to hydration and pH, a schedule that permits a larger amount of rest and convalescence than would (falsely believed to) be necessary with the ingestion of OTC drugs or suppressive medications. Although in our case, a motivating factor to find alternatives to those choices was that our allergies did not end with food. Both Alexandra and myself are highly allergic to many preservatives, colorings, and additives that would be present in many products, so there is an even greater risk for worse symptoms.

Alexandra's immune system has been maturing and strengthening over the years, and we attribute that to good choices. There was a time that even the slightest sneeze would create the need for her body to produce a fever to fight off the germ. In addition, her system responds to an inhaled allergen, (yes, she is allergic to many animals, scents, etc.) the same way as it would a virus. Years ago, not only would she catch colds so very easily, but it would take her two or three times as long as another child to recover and then rebound. There were very long periods of convalescence in her earlier years. Still today, she gets sick very easily, but the length of time of healing has decreased and her rebound time has improved greatly. She has recovered from several severe illnesses over the years with the aid of Fravarti and her expertise with homeopathy. Only once was Alexandra simply unable to endure the cure, and we consulted her pediatrician only to have a very tense few days trying desperately to find an antibiotic that did not produce severe allergic symptoms. The risk of antibiotic resistant bacteria production during this search was high, and we were extremely fearful; thankfully on the third attempt we landed on a drug she tolerated better and she responded. Of course the fall out afterward included a kidney infection. Another motivating factor in not reaching for drugs: we have genetic kidney issues that would make those organs a likely target for damage.

While we have practiced these beliefs over the years, it has become quite apparent that there is a life or death risk at hand. Therefore, we are not so foolish as to ignore the gifts of modern medicine that would have the potential to save Alexandra's life if need be. She carries an EpiPen, and while we always reach for Rescue Remedy first, second would be a homeopathic remedy if she doesn't respond, and if that didn't help either, the EpiPen would be next. Consequences of administering that drug might arise, but at least her life might be spared.

Educational choices are always a factor when you have a child who has limitations. She began in a small Christian school, and they were wonderful about accommodating her needs and working with us when she needed to be home. As she aged, though, and there were larger demands, school became difficult. Prolonged illnesses created difficulties and she was always catching something. We elected to bring her home to school early in third grade. We enjoyed home schooling for five years. She loved school and was very instrumental in maintaining academic excellence and a rigorous learning environment. While we participated in co-ops and extra-curricular activities, they were only when it suited her health. It was a wonderful experience and she was blessed with continued strengthening and healing. The long list of allergens began to shrink down. Sadly, she is Celiac like her father, so gluten will always be a no-no, but there were many foods which we were able to reintroduce in time, through occasionally challenge testing her.

Alexandra loved and missed a school environment, and our prayer was that she would be healthy enough to consider re-entry into high school. In seventh grade, a school came to our attention and it seemed like a good fit for her. We investigated and she began attending a University Model School in her eighth grade year. The students attend classes Monday, Wednesday, and Friday, and school at home independently the remainder of the week. Her work ethic and passion for learning made this set up a perfect match, and we were blessed to have been led to the precise courses during our home school years that allowed her to slide right in to her grade level.

Fast forward to Alexandra at age 16. She is a bright, creative, lively, passionate young lady. Does she still have to make difficult choices to achieve tolerable health? Absolutely. Does she still get sick easily? Yes, but she rebounds more quickly. Of course Celiac rarely ends with avoidance of gluten, and the autoimmune nature of the illness creates stress on the immune system and there is always a risk of other autoimmune diseases, so maintaining good health by great choices is an over-riding goal. At this age, we are trying to allow her liberties in making her own choices. With those choices, though, come consequences; so, we are all learning that it is still quite mandatory that she adhere to the protocols that we have been working through over the years. Rather than reach for drugs when she is under the weather, she gets into an Epsom Salts bath with wonderfully healing essential oils. She ramps up her supplementation of Vitamin C and other supportive supplements. She clears her calendar. While we frequently eat soups made with homemade protein broth, in these situations they become daily regimens and even drinking the broth straight up (if there is bronchial distress, she will fast on broth and we will incorporate Castor Oil packs to draw out congestion). Ultra hydration becomes an even higher priority, and of course absolutely no junk food, (this includes processed breads, pastas, and crackers). A diet to maintain a proper PH for her includes a large amount of raw fruits and vegetables, healthy proteins, and lots of filtered and structured water. Alexandra also manages her blood sugar with frequent meals which include healthy protein and a raw goodie.

Our prayer is that Alexandra will continue to strengthen and heal with good choices. Forcing her body to tolerate everything ranging from scents to foods she should not be eating, pushing beyond her physical capacity, and trying to keep up with a generation who gains their identity based on how many activities they can squeeze into a week, will all work against her. These choices become more and more difficult as she gets older. While we can see clearly that we, as parents, are also being given an opportunity to personally model for Alexandra what it looks like to put our personal and family needs first, it is extremely counter cultural. Being willing to make choices for your health will make you unpopular at times, and even offend some, but it is a journey we have willingly signed up for. It is an absolute joy to raise Alexandra, our severely allergic child, who has brought more happiness to our family then we could ever imagine.

FLU PREVENTION AND AWARENESS

I recall the earliest media announcements of the emergence of swine flu in Mexico. Newspaper coverage mentioned that the original outbreak occurred in an impoverished inner city barrio that had no pure, clean, safe water. The infection appeared to spread due to unsanitary conditions that the people had no power over. This flu was predicted to be potentially on course to reach epidemic proportions, at least in some areas.

Is it preventable? On an individual and family basis, the answer, in many cases, is yes. Can we keep it from sweeping through our communities and temporarily disabling large numbers of the most vulnerable? Maybe not, or at least, it will be difficult in some situations.

Who are the most vulnerable to this year's flu? Those with an acidic pH of 5.1 to 6.2 will be very vulnerable. Those whose hydration reads negative will be extremely vulnerable, as will those whose toxic burdens read above 5. By keeping the body's vital statistics within sustainable parameters for natural health and healing, we provide the best natural defense - a strong and resilient immune system. A urine pH above 6.5, together with optimal hydration (+7) and a low toxic burden (below 3 on a 10 point scale) allow the body to fend off infectious diseases with little or no pathology or symptoms. Those who are dehydrated and at lower urine pH levels, due to an acid forming diet of processed foods together with prescription and non-prescription medicines, are the most likely to develop severe symptoms and recover slowly.

To support the immune system, I recommend elderberry syrup, a supplement which is safe even for children and the elderly. For those who are the most compromised, I often recommend up to 2 tablespoons three times a day (in water) for two or three weeks. Many companies make a good elderberry syrup but for economy of price relative to a preventative dose over 2 or 3 weeks, Sambucus by Nature's Way is a wise choice. They also make Sambuguard, which is the same product with the addition of echinacea.

Vitamin C is also a good support for the immune system. Those wishing to build up their immunity can use 2 to 3 grams up to three times a day for two or three weeks. The adrenals, which are the largest user and concentration of vitamin C in the body, respond more resiliently to life's stresses when well supplied with this important nutrient (which in vibrational medicine, has the frequency of kindness and consideration).

Children through age 12 are considered to have higher risk of contracting the flu or of developing more severe symptoms for several reasons. One reason, in some cases, is the plethora of childhood vaccines - up to 27 immunizations in the first 24 months of life. Some of these children now have only half the health they started with and could still have, if the immunization schedule were changed dramatically and some vaccines eliminated.

Second, the children are dehydrated. America's school children rarely drink water and they mostly consume a diet of highly refined, processed foods which create an acid pH in the body and keep it from the healing influence of a higher or more optimal pH above 6.5. Over a period of years, the acid pH interferes with the acetylcholine cycle of the brain and interferes with cognitive functions such as focus and memory. If these children are put on psychiatric medicines to compensate for their inattention and resultant behavior problems, then the dehydration and acid pH become even more chronically disruptive and they develop anxiety and chronic illness as well as increasingly dysfunctional behaviors.

Children who drink 6 or more glasses of pure water daily and consume about 40% raw food will have a pH that is significantly higher (6.6 to 6.8) than children eating only processed foods and drinks. This higher pH protects us from many illness, both acute and chronic, including the flu, cancer, diabetes and dementia.

How do I feel about the flu vaccines? Flu shots have never been recommended in the intuitive readings. A killed attenuated virus vaccine may be better than a live virus nasal vaccine. The live virus could ultimately be instrumental in spreading the flu in certain vulnerable people. This has been known to happen with other live virus vaccines including polio.

For those who are most vulnerable, I prefer to use more natural methods of flu prevention including super-hydrating with pure water, maintaining proper alkaline pH range with a healthy diet of raw whole foods rather than a diet of convenience and processed foods together with the use of well indicated, safe, effective supplements. These could include elderberry syrup, vitamin C, oregano oil, GSE, and ashwaganda.

Oscillococcinum may reduce the severity of symptoms by as much as 50% or more if taken because of exposure to the flu, before symptoms develop. AirBorn may be effective for some people to protect against the flu. It may help promote resistance to bacterial throat infections when used before the symptoms are well developed.

To protect yourself from illness this season and next, drink 10 or more cups of pure structured water daily or drink Penta water. Eat raw food that is unprocessed: not Kashi cereal and Amy's enchiladas or rice bread, but rather whole fruit, vegetables, raw nuts and seeds, sprouts and greens, unprocessed meats and organic dairy.

Eat foods that are natural, not foods that say "Natural" on the package. This creates a more alkaline pH that protects us from viral infections and allows us to heal quickly. Include a proper balance of rest, relaxation and recuperation on a regular basis. Don't let hectic schedules and expectations take over. Find joy in doing less but don't overlook the importance of regular exercise and physical fitness.

Another healthy habit to develop is to avoid eating from open containers of food, particularly in grocery stores but also other large gatherings or parties. Any person passing by breathes their illness into the air which will be settling on open dishes of food like laboratory petri dishes designed to culture bacteria and disease. Sugary dishes such as punch bowls, cakes and candy are the most dangerous, but if a food server or food handler is sick, the risk is high no matter what the food. Stay home if you are sick: don't go to work, school or social events. Keep only health care related appointments until you are no longer contagious and encourage your family, friends and co-workers to do the same.

Regular hand washing, on average 7 to 9 times a day, is a highly effective measure of prevention. When used frequently, after each likely exposure, such as the use of a public restroom, hand washing can reduce exposure to illness by up to 85%. The voice of intuition provides frequent guidance and warnings to help us create optimum health if we are paying attention. Promptings to wash our hands, not stand close, or avoid certain foods come to us through feelings and sensations, magnetisms and attractions and repulsions, through color, sound, texture and smell. If we accept these wisdom messages from the body and the deeper knowing of intuition, we often avoid falling prey to whatever is going around.

Aromatherapy: doTerra OnGuard.

DIGESTIVE HEALTH

What is digestive health and why it is both cause and cure of so many maladies? Digestive health reflects the quality of nutrition, the quality of the environmental stresses, and even the quality of inherited constitutional weaknesses. About 70% of the immune functions begin in the gut. Not only does the abdomen contain numerous lymph nodes to provide immune system support because many illnesses enter the body through the mouth and stomach but also throughout the small intestines are cells called Peyer's Patches that have immune functions helping the body recognize and eliminate toxins and disease. Most allergies are a response of this part of the immune system, even those which are experienced as pollen related. One of the most extreme examples of digestive health as the source of allergies is called leaky gut syndrome.

When the mucosal covering of the microvilli of the small intestines becomes worn away deeply enough to expose the lymphatic vessels they contain, the contents of the gut then come into direct contact with immune cells that they are not meant to be in contact with. This triggers a hyper immune reaction of generalized misery in response to eating as the body becomes progressively more allergic to every bite you eat until the lining of the intestines is healed. Irritable Bowel Syndrome, Inflammatory Bowel Syndrome and Crohn's disease are all forms of leaky gut and can produce extremely disabling symptoms.

The combination of processed and convenience foods together with the chronic high stress life style that these fake foods are meant to ease or at least make possible has created some form of bowel disease for over 100 million Americans. Those symptoms can be brought under control and those digestive systems returned to health when we acknowledge the body's message that this essential system is not working well and make changes to meet the body's real needs. The gut is not only a messenger of our moods through the enteric nervous system but it is also influencing and regulating our moods through the production of serotonin in the stomach lining. A food journal that includes not only what you ate but why you did so and how you felt can be very empowering. We are a nation of stress eaters, binge eaters and sugar addicts often consuming 50% of our calories as non-nutritive fake foods.

We do need comfort foods that increase our experience of emotional fulfillment, but we can choose healthier comfort foods by making them from scratch from wholesome ingredients. The body needs about 30% protein, 30% healthy fats and less that 15% sugars. That leaves 25% to 30% for complex carbohydrates. The body needs a specific pH range of 6.6 to 6.8, and it needs optimum hydration. Digestion alone takes a couple gallons of water per day.

Due to the water conservation function of the large intestine, most of that water in the digestive system is retained. Only about 1/2 cup will be lost through the bowel movements. It is because of this water recovery function of the colon that humans and animals are able to live on dry land. If the bowels become sluggish and delayed in emptying, more water may be reabsorbed from the feces waiting to exit the colon and this will produce constipation and hard dry stools. This calls for some form of extra support for the sluggish bowel which might include probiotics, digestive enzymes, magnesium, possibly a gentle herbal stimulant like Dr. Miller's Holy Tea, and even abdominal massage in the direction of intestinal flow. Sluggish digestion and sluggish bowels can also be improved by regular exercise. Walking, biking, yoga, trampoline, dance and hula-hoop are all good choices to create more core strength and ease of digestion.

Digestion is about supplying glucose for the brain and nutrients for every cell of the body. Obesity results when those basic needs of the body are not met because the hunger message is not turned off by the consumption of non-nutritive fake foods. Even when the digestive system is on overload, it will still register hunger if it lacks needed nutrients.

Studies have shown that the consumption (before and during a meal) of a 44 oz. beverage sweetened with HFCS does not reduce the amount of calories consumed at that meal, because the brain cannot use HFCS and so does not register as being fed and therefore does not release the appetite suppressing hormone leptin. The HFCS will be processed by the liver, and when there is an excess or more than can be eliminated, it will be stored as fat, both in the liver as an undesirable phenomena called fatty liver, and as abdominal fat, accumulating and forming belly fat. HFCS does not feed you, but it does make you fat. The body stores accumulated toxins in fat, so not only does the body not look the way we prefer, the feeling of generalized un-wellness, queezy, uneasy gut, nausea, cramping, bloating, and all manner of abdominal distress, as well as generalized physical distress, weakness, and even headache, dizzy spells or fainting can result from this toxic burden that is being stored instead of efficiently excreted by the overtaxed systems of the body. One of the toxins that gets stored and accumulates in the body of those who consume HFCS is glyphosate. Also known as the herbicide Round Up, glyphosate is sprayed on the GMO corn crop twice in its growing season. It is assimilated into the plant cells and passed on to those who eat those crops, including livestock as well as humans.

The liver and gall bladder are responsible for regulating fat metabolism. The liver makes bile, which breaks down fats, and the gallbladder stores bile and releases it into the small intestine. Gallbladder removal is one of the most common surgeries in America. When gallstones are present or a constriction of the bile duct is diagnosed, removal of the organ is recommended with seeming casual disregard for what has caused the stones or stricture. Eliminating highly refined processed foods from the diet, (particularly those made with unhealthy oils) together with eliminating fried foods, reduces gallstone build up and the acute flare ups of abdominal pain which indicate that the gallbladder has become inflamed and possibly infected. In the tradition of Oriental Medicine, healing the gallbladder, instead of removing it, is the first step towards improved liver health and greater optimism in the mental emotional out look.

The body needs fats. The brain needs healthy fats such as raw nuts and avocados. No part of the body needs fried oils, rancid oils or trans-fats such as margarine.

Protect your body's ability to assimilate and metabolize omega fatty acids that you need by not overtaxing these organs with toxic non-nutritive fats like canola oil. American canola oil contains glyphosate because it is a GMO crop designed for use with this herbicide which lingers in the cells of the plant and is now being found in breast milk in America's nursing mothers. Eating healthy fats supports weight loss. The fats that promote acute gallbladder episodes also promote obesity.

Insulin resistance and the resultant type 2 diabetes that it produces are, at their onset, reversible diseases that can be healed. At some point many years after that onset, diabetes is considered no longer reversible. Diabetics who are assisted by conventional modern medicines today are not expected to ever get better and maintaining them on life long medication is actually the goal of their treatment. Eating a diet that causes the blood sugar to spike at levels above 150 regularly and then reducing blood sugar levels with medication is called managing diabetes. Using this approach to symptom management always results in the worsening of the severity of the diabetes and eventually leads to one or more of the other consequences of advancing diabetes which include: increased risk of heart disease, stroke, high blood pressure, kidney disease, blindness, dementias, neuropathy and amputation of limbs.

Omega 3 fats have the effect of improving the body's response to insulin and it's ability to restore and maintain normal blood sugar levels. Insomnia specifically increases insulin resistance and promotes obesity. Lowering the stress level to support healthy sleep cycles is a significant factor of any protocol meant to address the cause that weakens digestive health and promote diabetes and pre-diabetes known as insulin resistance.

Heartburn and esophageal reflux also result from frequent consumption of a diet that is not well matched to your body's needs and digestive abilities. Digestive functions weaken when the diet consistently contains more of what harms the body than it contains of that which is beneficial. This failure to balance consumption more sustainably has emotional and social/cultural underpinnings. The modern American diet is a response to other factors that don't work in our lives, including ever increasing stress and a cultural shift away from spending time preparing food.

Maintaining a therapeutic diet designed to heal disease and restore health can take about one third of your life devoted to holding the concentration of eating sustainably. If you have enough financial freedom to hire personal chefs and buy from local raw food chefs and farmers markets to supplement what you make yourself, you can still devote plenty of time to both work and play and consistently eat healthy and sustainably. If you can't afford to pay someone to make your raw nut milks, bliss balls, raw pies and fresh raw juice, then you will need to re-configure how you spend your time to allow for eliminating convenience foods and making fresh homemade from whole unprocessed foods. Your life truly does depend on it and so does the quality of the life you experience each day.

Long term medication with acid reducing drugs that allow you to continue to consume a diet that clearly is not working for you will undermine not only your daily experience of physical wellness but also undermine your cognitive functions, effectively reducing both clarity of thought and comprehension as well as reducing memory functions. The need for acid reducing medications is a warning from the intelligent operating systems of the body. It is not a warning that you need to take medication for the rest of your life while the symptoms persist or worsen. It is a message that the contents of the gut do not support wellness and that patterns of consumption, including amounts, ingredients and styles of preparation all need to be evaluated as possible promoters of this problem. Medication for short term acute relief should quickly be replaced with more sustainable choices. These medications should not be continued year after year to allow for continued consumption of those food addictions which become our substitute for the life we really need to create for ourselves and loved ones.

Bowel Disease

Constipation, hemorrhoids, inflammation, candida, parasites, Leaky Gut Syndrome, IBS, colitis, Crohn's, Gastoesophogeal reflux, food allergies

Spiritual / Emotional:

Negative self-image, Self-pity, Martyr.

Symptoms:

Abdominal cramps, pain, bloating, gas, heartburn, constipation, diarrhea, hemorrhoids.

Causes:

Antibiotics and other prescription medications, Candida overgrowth, diet lacking whole foods, excessive consumption of convenience foods, fake foods, highly refined processed foods, Nutrasweet (Aspartame), chocolate, unhealthy oils, corn syrup, alcohol, caffeine, dehydration, acidosis, obesity, sedentary lifestyle, hypo-thyroid, pesticide exposure.

Treatments:

Whole fresh foods. Organic only!
Elimination diet - canola, soybean oil, cottonseed oil, margarine, hydrogenated oils, rancid oils, chocolate, corn syrup, sodas, wheat, soy, oranges, pork, processed meats, alcohol, coffee, all processed grains, dairy
Candida diet (90 days), Raw Food diet (120 days), Celiac diet, Rotation diet, or modified fasting
Broth - 3 cups per day
Fresh Ginger Tea - 5 cups per day.
Peppermint tea Hydration - 10 cups of structured water daily

Colonics, enemas, basti - (4 oz. flax oil)
Edgar Cayce Castor Oil packs over abdomen every 3 days x 40 repetitions of 3 hours
Exercise 60 minutes per day 6 x week, increases intestinal motility.
Trampoline

Supplements And Botanicals:

Massage - Deep Tissue or Rolfing
Flax seed, fresh ground - 3 tsp. daily
Slippery Elm - 2 capsules 3 x day
Triphala - 2,000 mgs 3 x day x 3 months
Probiotics, mixed - 3 x day
Green Vibrance - fights yeast and supports detoxing
Digestive Enzymes - 3 x day, supports pancreas and duodenum
Black walnut tincture - 3 droppers 3 x day, parasite cleanse - roundworms
Artemesia, wormwood - 1,000 mgs 2 x day - pinworms
Oregano Oil by Gaia - 2 caps per dose up to 3 x day (with meals) - tapeworm
Vitamin C - 2 grams 3 x day
Colon Clenz - herbal combination for occasional use for relief of constipation
Candidagone - herbal support for candida cleanse
Dr. Miller's Holy Tea - for relief of bloating and sluggish bowel. Heals the large intestine
Quercetin - fast acting, short acting relief from symptoms caused by food allergies
Essiac - support for cancer recovery
doTerra Ginger oil
Kombucha - fresh sourced, not bottled commercially (for diarrhea) Zeolite
Detoxamin - EDTA suppositories
Counseling, therapy and support groups for emotional eating and food trauma issues
* Discontinue vitamins and some supplements during parasite cleanse (parasites eat them)

BONE HEALTH

United States Surgeon General Dr. Richard Carmona warned that 50% of Americans will face serious bone health issues due to lifestyle and habits that put them at risk. Poor nutrition together with sedentary pastimes instead of physical activity significantly reduce bone health. Our acid-forming diets cause the minerals calcium and magnesium to be pulled from our bones and teeth and returned to the blood stream to buffer the acidosis and restore more normal pH. Because vitamin D3 is used to transport these minerals back out of bones and teeth to buffer the pH, the body is now using much more vitamin D than it requires in a normal state of optimum pH. Sunlight is a primary promoter of healthy levels of vitamin D in the body but many Americans have come to consider sunlight as something to be avoided. An active lifestyle that includes regular exercise, particularly weight bearing exercise (which includes walking), as well as stretching, builds bone strength and resilience.

The skeleton and the health of all tissues related to it are profoundly affected by the health of the kidneys. Rebuilding bone health always means restoring kidney health as the foundation for recovery of bone strength and resilience and bones need both strength to hold our bodies up without pain and resilience to prevent fractures from normal activities and minor accidents. Strength and resilience are two different factors of bone health, and modern prescription drugs designed to increase bone strength have been shown to reduce bone resilience over time and result in fractures that would not occur in truly healthy bone. The solution lies in restoring the body's ability to make healthy bones by providing for the body's real needs to restore health to the deep core of our constitutional vitality through optimum hydration, a diet which produces alkaline pH in the body's tissue, and an active lifestyle that includes regular exercise together with stress reducing choices to maintain physical and psychological balance. A weakness of bone health is a weakness of the deep constitutional health and will be successfully resolved only when addressed holistically by restoring health to the whole being.

One's self concept is also held in the core of the body as well as in the core of one's being. That self image shapes and informs the body's strengths and weaknesses. The minerals calcium and magnesium, essential for formation of healthy bones, hold the frequencies of safety, confidence, security, and even courage. The pulling of these minerals from bones and teeth to buffer acidosis is usually accompanied by a conscious awareness of increasing anxiety and worry that is rapidly and noticeably relieved by taking these minerals in a form that is easy for the body to assimilate. Rebuilding strength and resilience in one's self image is part of developing a strong core for the physical body. The very same substance and lifestyle choices that weaken every part of the human body consistently in all cases, are the things which eventually deplete bone health and lead to bone diseases and bone failures. Smoking, alcohol, drugs and Rx medications, high stress, acidosis, dehydration, malnutrition, caffeine and obesity all increases the burden on the kidneys, accelerate aging processes and promote general weakening of all organs and systems from memory to eyesight and hearing while silently and perhaps unnoticed, the bones are giving up their life and vitality to try to meet the demands of an unnatural life. Our bones are strongest between age 20 and 30, but they constitute a storehouse of vital strength that can be rapidly depleted when continuously challenged and overtaxed by our choices in life. It is not as rapid a process to rebuild bone health and remineralize teeth and bones as it is to lose it. It can take two years or more to reverse deteriorating bone health.

Bones

The ability to stand up for oneself. Resentment.

Osteoporosis

Losing bone mass and density, bones become brittle, due to demineralization.

Causes:

Low progesterone, chronic dehydration and acidosis pulling calcium from the bones to buffer the acid pH.
Soft drinks, processed foods, sugar, alcohol, coffee, caffeine, fluoride. Kidney disease. Inadequate fluid intake.
Thyroid hormone calcitonin maintains proper calcium levels for healthy bones.

Treatments:

Raw juice - 3 cups daily to raise pH
ProGest Cream twice daily, liberal use
Calcium 1,000 mgs daily, coral calcium, raw calcium,
Floradix liquid calcium, whole food sourced calcium, carrots, greens

Vitamin K - 300 mgs 2x day
Folic Acid 800 mcgs. and Vitamin B 100 complex
Sam-e, sadenosyl methionine
Kelp, MSM, Black Cohosh
Water - 10 or more cups per day of structured water
Probiotics, bifidus
Vitamin C
Fresh ginger tea
Broth - 2 cups per day, especially marrow broth or bone broth
GLA - black currant or evening primrose oil
Osteopathic adjustments
Osteoclasts breakdown old bone. Osteoblasts create new bone. Boniva and Fosamax increase bone mass at the expense of resilience leading to hip fractures after 5 years

Osteoarthritis

Affects 40 to 50 million Americans. The most common type of arthritis due to wear and tear, mechanical destruction, injury and hard use of joints. Most common locations - fingers, knees, hips, neck and lumbar spine. Cartilage breaks down and bones rub against bone, especially in large weight bearing joints and in the hands.

Treatments:

Castor Oil Packs
GLA, Evening Primrose Oil - 3,000 mgs daily
Fish Oils - Nordic Naturals ProOmega 4,000 mgs daily, doTERRA - xEO Mega 4,000 mgs daily
B 100 complex
Calcium - 1,000 mgs daily or 2 caps 2 x day
Probiotics - bifidus, Udo's Super 8 Selenium - 200 mcgs 2x day
MSM - 2 grams twice a day
Fresh ginger tea - anti-inflammatory, raises pH
Exercise 60 minutes per day 6 days a week. Weight bearing exercise increases bone health.
Osteopathic adjustments.
Rolfing
Homeopathic - Rhus Tox, Staphysagria
Bone Broth - beef or chicken broth cooked with bones in, marrow broth
Raw juice
Vitamin E

Rheumatoid Arthritis

Affects about 2 million Americans, mostly women. Fibromyalgia is also rheumatism. Inflammatory auto-immune disease. Suppressed infection. Occurs mostly in the small joints, synovial membranes become swollen, red and hot. Disease process lays down scar tissue in the joints.

Other Causes:

Smoking, antibiotics, heavy metal toxicity, pesticides, food allergies (in 60% of cases, esp. tomato, dairy and sugar).
Fasting and general detox and cleansing is supportive

Treatments:

Selenium - 200 mcgs 2 x a day
Vitamin C - 2 to 4 grams per day
Copper - 3 mgs
Folic Acid - 800 mcgs Calcium - 1,000 mgs daily
Fish Oils Nordic Natural ProOmega - 2,000 mgs 2 x day, doTERRA - xEO Mega - 2,000 mgs 2 x day
Probiotics, bifidus
Fresh Ginger Tea Exercise
Osteopathic adjustments
Meditation and relaxation techniques
Neuromuscular massage. Reflexology.
Homeopathic - Bryonia, worse slightest movement.
Staphysagria, suppressed disease.
*   Avoid antacids containing aluminum

KIDNEYS

The kidneys, together with the adrenals, reflect the state of the core of your being. The kidney adrenal complex (adrenal means top of the kidney) is comprised of two organs which sit one on each side, right and left of the spine at about the waist and slightly above. The adrenal complex is the body's store house of chi or vital energy and when depleted of this vital core energy, the body's health manifests the symptoms of its weakness as blood pressure problems, failing bone health, infertility, hair loss and a mental emotional outlook of fear and inadequacy. Restoring health and vitality to one's core is essential to recovering and maintaining health in any and all of the other organs and systems of the body. Current published estimates indicate that more than 26 million Americans have chronic kidney disease and that one in three of us are at risk for developing kidney disease. Cases of kidney disease are increasing rapidly in our modern culture of dehydration and acidosis and the primary causal factors are diet, chemicals, drugs and stress.

Primary functions of the kidneys are filtering all water soluble toxins from the body's fluids and maintaining blood pH at an alkaline 7.364. Modern life has exponentially increased the burden on the kidneys by increasing the number and amount of toxins to be filtered, reducing the intake of pure water and lowering the pH in the kidneys to a state of chronic acidosis. The lower the pH is below 7, the harder the kidneys are working to maintain critical blood pH and the sooner they become weakened. To take the burden off of the kidneys and allow them to heal, it is essential to optimize hydration and pH in the body by maintaining a therapeutic diet designed to raise pH, by elimination of processed foods, (especially grains), and consuming large amounts of raw foods.

Strengthening the core through exercise and attaining an optimal weight range and waist measurement are also necessary to create and maintain kidney health. Obesity increases the burden on the kidneys and is a risk factor for chronic kidney weakness. Core strength and health in the kidney adrenal complex promotes confidence, courage and optimism in the psyche.

Kidney weakness and Kidney Disease

Symptoms:

Swelling - around the eyes, the feet, legs and hands. Bad taste in mouth, odor in breath, increasing blood pressure, dry, itchy skin, anxiety, shortness of breath, and hair loss.
Contributing factors include: Mold allergy, uric acid, diabetes, insulin resistance, hypertension, osteoporosis, hair loss, eczema, nail fungus

Causes:

Alcohol, pesticide, dehydration, inadequate fluid intake. Habitually drinking everything but water - such as coffee, soda, juice. High sugar diet and highly processed wheat.

Issue:

Fear, inadequacy, criticism and fear of criticism, praise and blame, rejection, unloveable.

Natural Therapies:

Adequate hydration is key to recovery. Increase water to 10 cups daily. Use Structured water. Avoid alcohol, caffeine (including over the counter meds), all soft drinks, sugar and refined flours. Dietary changes are necessary to manage chronic kidney weakness. Vegetarian, blood type diet, fasting and modified fasting (broth and ginger infusion) are all recommended
Exercise
Massage, foot reflexology

Supplements:

Magnesium - Natural Calm by Natural Vitality is the fastest most effective magnesium supplement.
Vitamin C - 3 x day, 2 grams per dose
Complete omega's
Vitamin E - 800 I.U.'S
Shiitake mushrooms - 3,000 mgs
Bach Flowers - including Sweet Chestnut for emotional anguish
Kneipp Lavender Bath 4 to 6 times per week

Ginger Root - Fresh homemade ginger root tea can be served hot, cold, or room temperature. 3 or more cups per day
Lemon Juice - Edgar Cayce gentle kidney cleanse is 8 oz. lemon water, 8 times a day made with 1/2 fresh squeezed lemon per glass or 3 to 4 lemons per day
Raw Juice - 3 cups daily to restore hydration and pH
Watermelon
Conscious relaxation to reduce stress, balance
Exercise to increase stamina and resilience

ADRENALS

Getting it all done, catching up and keeping up all take a toll on the adrenals. A very demanding pace that pushes us to do and accomplish at maximum levels every day depletes us of stamina and resilience, by overtaxing the adrenals and sending the body into a 'fight or flight' mode. Over scheduling, commitments and expectations that are often unrealistic as well as unhealthy. Cortisol flooding in response to the judgement of not good enough and not getting enough done or done right is the modern cultural tiger chasing the modern man, woman and child through a landscape of criticism and blame.

We try to be good enough by relentlessly doing all that we can in the way of self improvement and accomplishments every day, but it's never enough and we reach deep exhaustion long before we could ever reach the illusion of getting it all done, caught up, and done well enough to gain the much desired validation that we are seeking with this persistent efforting. Adrenal exhaustion and adrenal failure are produced by a relentless assault on the coping mechanisms of the body and an unrelenting state of overwhelm in which the body's real needs go unmet. Even the psyche's real needs go unmet because the contract that you will get a break when it's all done is never fulfilled.

You try as hard as you can but... it's never enough. There is always more to do and do right now or right away. The timing, the pace, the pressure are all artificial, unnatural and maintained only at a price, a physical toll on the body mind experience that leaves one weakened, frantic, frustrated and less and less capable. Adrenal exhaustion is a factor in fibromyalgia, migraine, pneumonia, lyme's disease, bi-polar depression, PTSD and many other states of "burn out".

To restore adrenal health, strength and resilience can be both slow and challenging. Part of the support system is convincing your adrenals that you are lying in a hammock sipping lemonade, on vacation, so to speak, and they are not needed. Lots of intentionally doing nothing or as little as possible, lots of silence and personal space and no stress, ever, are the parameters that support adrenal recovery. Meditation, prayer, journaling, yoga, the quietest, calmest activities that conserve or create energy in the core of your being will produce resilience and adaptability in time.

Adrenal Exhaustion

30 million Americans have some form of adrenal insufficiency.

Symptoms:

Debilitating weakness and fatigue not relieved by rest or sleep, which is disabling of basic daily activities including work, play, self care and exercise. Poor temperature regulation, sensitivities to both hot and cold. Lymphatic swellings, hormone deficiencies, dysbiosis and intestinal parasites. Adrenal exhaustion is a factor in fibromyalgia. It's pain is due to accumulation of uric acid. Chronic fatigue syndrome is a form of adrenal failure.

Causes:

Physical burnout, excessive work. Unhealthy diet of high fructose corn syrup and refined flours. Medications (especially steroids and anxiety medications) P.T.S.D., Bi-polar disorder, chronic acute illness (including pneumonia, Lyme's and Mono).

Issues:

Willingness to be balanced, to listen to the body respectfully and observe healthy rhythms of rest and activity. Doing instead of being. Achievement as false self esteem. Over Responsible.

Natural Therapies:

High protein broth - 3 cups daily
Raw food diet, Raw Juice - 3 cups daily
Vitamin B100 complex
Vitamin C - 3 x day, 3 grams per dose.
   * The adrenal glands use vitamin C at a higher rate than any other cells. The need rises in response to stress. The adrenals are the largest user and largest storehouse of vitamin C in the body. I.V. vitamin C may be necessary in states of collapse. Vitamin C has the frequency of kindness.
Elderberry Syrup - 1 tablespoon in water 3 x day

Floradix Floravital - gluten free liquid vitamin / iron formula
5 HTP - up to 300 mgs daily
CoQ10 - 300 to 400 mgs 2 x day, CoQ10 protects the brain from cortisol
Alpha lipoic acid - 600 mgs 2 x a day
Colostrum
Valerian - 400 mgs at night
Rescue Remedy in Structured water - 6 droppers full in each of 2 or more liters daily
Cordyceps mushrooms
Edgar Cayce Castor oil packs, every 2 to 4 days for 30 repetitions of 2 to 4 hours each
ProGest cream for menopausal and premenopausal women
Kneipp Lavender baths 6 days a week
Epsom salts baths
Neuro-muscular massage and Lymphatic drainage massage
Yoga exercise and Chi Gong
Reduce activity level by 20% (but maintain moderate exercise, walking, stretching)
Increase silence to 4 hours daily
Journaling, practices of self-examination
Personal Retreats, half day mini-retreats, 3 day retreats, 10 day retreat or longer

THYROID

Located at the base of the throat in front of the wind pipe, this small organ influences metabolic processes throughout the body. The production of hormones by the thyroid is based on iodine chemistry. If thyroid hormone level is low, the thyroid will enlarge in an attempt to concentrate more iodine in thyroid tissue. That enlargement of the thyroid gland is called goiter and is very responsive to iodine supplementation. Thyroid hormones regulate oxygen uptake in the cells of the body and regulate temperature.

The thyroid also regulates the breakdown of fats and cholesterol for the production of energy. That production of energy is called metabolism. Thyroid weakness causes a sluggish metabolism, weight gain, low energy and weak concentration. For proper regulation of the body's oxygen levels, heart rate, temperature and energy, thyroid hormones must be within a specific range. Excess of thyroid hormone causes as much disruption in the body as deficient hormone levels and produces a state of restless nervousness, jittery and shaky and increased appetite, possibly with weight loss.

The production of thyroid hormone (T4) is regulated by the pituitary gland in the brain. Thyroid hormone is then converted in the body (outside the thyroid) by the action of enzymes to its active form (T3) which acts as a stimulant throughout the body. Each of these three factors, thyroid stimulation hormone from the brain, production of hormones by the thyroid, and conversion in the body of the thyroid hormone to its active form, is essential to thyroid health and metabolism.

Both Ayurvedic and Chinese Medicine focus on detoxing the body (panchakarma and bupleurum) and adjusting the diet to promote thyroid balance. Risk factors for thyroid weakness include nutritional deficiencies, heavy metal or chemical toxicity, chronic high stress and acidosis. High cortisol levels specifically disrupt several other hormones and specifically block the conversions of T4 to its active form T3. Both soy beans and peanuts are also known to interfere with the production of thyroid hormones. Raw Kale and raw cabbage also inhibit thyroid hormone production. Supplements for thyroid support are iodine, zinc, copper, tyrosine (an amino acid) and thyroid glandular tissue. Chlorine and fluoride interfere with normal iodine chemistry by blocking iodine receptors in the thyroid.

There is a direct correlation between thyroid health and bone health. Poor thyroid function weakens bone health. Contained within the thyroid gland is a second set of glands called the parathyroid glands. These tiny glands regulate calcium levels in the blood and stimulate osteoclasts in the bones. When the pH is acidic instead of alkaline, the parathyroids signal for minerals (calcium and magnesium) to be pulled from the bones and teeth in order to buffer the acidosis.

Issues:

Location throat. Disruption of the thyroid chemistry can produce anxiety and depression. Expression, voice, fearing others' opinions.

Natural Therapies:

For spiritual/physical healing - 45 minutes of singing 3 or more times per week 5 million Americans have thyroid weakness.

Most thyroid problems require professional medical evaluation and supervision even when pursuing natural healing. Through its hormones, the thyroid regulates all metabolic processes in the body including regulation of the body temperature (also adrenals), uptake of oxygen and metabolism (also pancreas and liver) and production of progesterone. Thyroid function is based on iodine chemistry as well as calcium regulation. Regular physical activity, including 60 minutes of exercise six days a week, is important to support production of thyroid hormone, improve thyroid function and reverse thyroid damage.

Normal thyroid tissue has a pH of 8.3. This is the highest pH in the body. Therefore, low pH markedly weakens thyroid health.

Most common types:

Hypothyroid

Under functioning thyroid produces cold, low body temp, sluggish, lethargic, weight gain - particularly abdominally, constipation, dry skin, puffy face.

Hashimoto's Thyroiditis

Hashimoto's Thyroiditis is an autoimmune disorder which causes the thyroid to produce anti-thyroid antibodies which gradually destroy the thyroid tissue and suppress its functions. Both celiac disease and non-celiac wheat sensitivity are factors that strongly predispose to the onset and advancement of this autoimmune disorder. Completely eliminating exposures to food allergies, including wheat, is essential to supporting the body in reducing or eliminating the anti-thyroid antibodies.

Many people discover that they have been experiencing the symptoms of this disease for years before finding out what is behind it. Common symptoms of this disorder reflect the under functioning thyroid as a primary weakness. Low energy, low mood, easy weight gain, temperature sensitivity or poor body temperature regulation, digestive weakness, hair loss (especially eyebrows) and even joint and muscle pain are all part of the symptom picture of this progressively deteriorating autoimmune disorder. Natural therapies include iodine supplements (and in some cases selenium or zinc) and a diet modified to raise pH above 6.6 while eliminating all probable allergens and triggers.

High stress can also be a factor in promoting Hashimoto's because stress uses up iodine stores more quickly as well as disrupting the hormone balance directly through elevated cortisol levels relative to the diminishing levels of other hormones.

Hyperthyroid

Promotes weight loss, increased appetite and thirst, anxiety, palpitations, infrequent menses.

Causes:

Iodine deficiency causes the thyroid to enlarge (goiter).
Pituitary deficiency of TSH (primary test).
Congenital deficiency.
Sedentary lifestyle, lack of activity.
Stress, including physical stress, produces high cortisol and disrupts hormone balance.

Acid forming diet.

Decreased potassium levels from lack of whole foods.

Weak liver. T4 converts to T3 in the liver. T3 stimulates all physiological functions.

Environmental toxins, Fluoride, caffeine, aspartame, lead, petroleum distilates and solvents, and general Toxic Overload with acid pH.

Treatments:

Raw juice to raise the pH to 6.8. (not Kale)

Eliminate wheat, all grains and processed foods to raise pH

Allopathic – Thyroxin (T4), Synthroid, radiation, surgery

Armour Thyroid - animal thyroid extract, full hormone spectrum

Wilson's Thyroid Px - 5 mgs of Iodine plus herbs

Metabolic Advantage by Enzymatic Therapy- iodine, zinc, copper, tyrosine (weight loss)

Michael's Thyroid Factors - iodine, moss, chromium, bladderwrack and tyrosine Thytropin PMG by Standard Process - 45 mgs bovine thyroid concentrate

Nutrients:

Tyrosine

Glutamine 250 mgs 2 times a day

Niacin (B3)

Iron (20 mgs a day)

Gaia Plant force Iron or Floradix Omegas-Essential

Fatty Acids - fish oil 2,000 mgs 2 x per day.

Kelp (contains iodine).

Liquid Iodine: Atomadine (by Edgar Cayce),
Biotic Research or Eidon Ionic Minerals

Botanicals:

Bupleurum for cleansing

Ashwaganda 500 mgs

Ginger root tea - 3 to 5 cups daily to change pH.

Parathyroids

Function is regulation of calcium. This hormone in the blood stimulates osteoclasts in the bone and stimulates the kidneys to retain calcium. Calcium levels play a role in hyperactivity, senile dementia, psychosis, and seizures, as well as the mineralization of teeth and bones.

LIVER

The liver is the largest (by volume) organ in the body and one of the most important for sustaining natural health. The liver has more than a dozen major functions in the regulation of metabolism and liver weakness is one of the most common ways for the human body to breakdown. The most common stressors including chemical and drug exposure, alcohol and tobacco use and a high sugar diet together with chronic high cortisol levels due to unrelenting stress. Liver failure is not currently medically diagnosable until liver function is diminished by 90%. Liver functions have been weakening and presenting the symptomology of the liverish state for a long time, in most cases, before being recognized. Liver inflammation from alcohol, drugs and disease cause fibrotic scarring of hepatic tissue that remains even after the liver regenerates as fully as possible.

A damaged liver stores fat and a fatty liver is functionally inefficient. The liver becomes congested, tender and inflamed, producing nausea, vomiting, abdominal pain and bloating, gas and colic and a very slow passage of matter through the complex of digestive organs. This also causes slower passage of nutrients into the blood supply and slower removal of toxins from the blood, which then over burdens other organs and systems. Brain function is effectively reduced as to cognitive abilities when it receives blood from the liver that is inadequately filtered and the toxic burden begins to be stored in the brain producing chronic problems with memory, clarity and learning as the chemistry in the brain is altered by the failing liver functions.

Functions of the liver include the production of hormones including T3 for thyroid and the production of enzymes particularly for emulsifying fats, the production of bile salts, the synthesis of proteins, production of red blood cells and clotting factors, detoxification processes to render toxins harmless and remove them from the body including the conversion of ammonia to urea. The liver stores glycogen (sugars) and fats and releases them as energy. The liver makes cholesterol from fatty acids and makes fatty acids for the brain from cholesterol as needed. The liver stores all fat soluble vitamins including Vitamins A, D, E, K and some B12. The liver also stores iron and copper for use in production of healthy blood.

Poor Liver Function

Symptoms of poor liver function: Nausea, diarrhea, constipation, abdominal bloating and pain, colic, gas, heartburn, sinus infections, parasites (round or pin worms), yeast overgrowth, significant weight gain mid-body, puffy face, rectal fissures, skin rashes and sores. Hepatitis C (5 million Americans), inflammatory bowel disease (this is not the immune system attacking the body, this is the diet attacking the body). Includes Crohn's Disease and ulcerative colitis.

Hypo-thyroid because the liver makes the thyroid hormone T3 that the thyroid converts to T4. The body needs exercise for metabolism and movement for intestinal function and lymph circulation. Type II diabetes, insulin resistance, Allergies.

Pesticide on the food creates liver weakness which produces allergies. Cholesterol - bad cholesterol is elevated by high fructose corn syrup

Causes:

Alcohol, caffeine (which is contained in many over the counter medications and drugs), coffee, sodas, artificial sweeteners, high fructose corn syrup, sugar, pesticide, drugs, hydrogenated oils, grains - wheat, corn and soy. Highly refined processed foods. Meat and dairy with growth hormones. All of these produce dehydration, sluggish liver function and escalating toxic burden in the body.

Hepatitis

Hepatitis means infection of the liver. The source can be bacterial, viral or toxic (drug or chemical). Most hepatitis is acute and recovery occurs within 6 months. Prolonged relapsing and chronic hepatitis can cause permanent damage including pervasive scarring of liver tissue called cirrhosis and also liver cancer. Only hepatitis due to toxins including drug and chemical poisoning is noninfectious.

Infectious hepatitis (including viral hepatitis A, B, C and D) are transmissible by fecal oral contamination through food, water, kissing, hand contamination (fingers to mouth or open sores), sharing razors, toothbrushes, drug and tattoo needles and unprotected sex. In about a third of all cases, the exact source is not known. Occurance of type B and C hepatitis increases significantly with high number of sexual partners. Type C can exist for years with no symptoms. Both type B and C can be contagious even when the carrier is unaware of the disease and does not feel sick.

Common symptoms include chronic nausea, physical weakness and both mental and physical exhaustion. Symptoms sometimes include fever, aching, bruising, bleeding and jaundice. These symptoms may persist for months or years. Up to 75% of those who contract type C hepatitis develop a chronic form that produces liver damage in the form of cirrhosis or liver cancer and in later stages manifests significant mental confusion and cognitive impairment. This chronic form continues to be contagious, especially during relapsing episodes.

Judicious hand washing is significant for protection from this common infection. Treatment for all types of hepatitis include extra rest, healthy diet, elimination of all drugs and alcohol and careful attention to hydration. For chronic and relapsing forms of hepatitis, weekly infusions of intravenous alpha lipoic acid are recommended to reverse and heal liver damage.

Issues:

Issues of Personal Power, Self Esteem, and Martyrdom

Natural Therapies:

Structured water, high protein broth, Ginger tea, liquid diet for assimilation of nutrients with minimal digestion of solids, Organic healing diet, no processed food, lots of greens including chlorella, barley green, basil for detoxing. Eliminate refined flours and whole meats (use broth). Blood Type Diet, Vegetarian Diet
Milk Thistle - (inflammatory bowel) 500 mgs daily,
Poke Root (ulcerative colitis)
Shiitake - 2,000 to 3,000 mgs daily
Fresh ginger and ginger tea
Floradix for malnutrition from malabsorption and Floradix with Iron for anemia
NAC - N-acetyl L-cysteine
Acidophilus, Ruteri,
Digestive enzymes - lipase, amylase, protease, lactase - for pancreas and digestion
Alpha lipoic Acid - 600 mgs 2 x a day for liver disease, or I.V. ALA therapy
Edgar Cayce Castor Oil Packs over liver, spleen, abdomen
Greens, barley green, chlorella, basil, watercress, spinach, cilantro
Omega 3 oils, flax oil for vegetarians
Black Walnut tincture - (parasites), also Paragone
Magnesium 500 mgs twice daily
Exclusion Diet - eliminate alcohol, OTC drugs, prescriptions, artificial sweeteners, wheat, corn, soy, chicken, chocolate, orange juice, coffee, sugar, processed foods. Failure to eliminate food, drug and alcohol factors results in continued reactivity and symptoms, escalating toxic levels

in the body due to chronic dehydration, falling vital force and weakened constitution. Nausea, bloating, uncomfortable. Pregnant look about the belly.

Exercise 60 minutes per day 5 days per week

Neuro-muscular Massage and Lymphatic Drainage Massage

ORAL AND DENTAL HEALTH

The overall health of the individual greatly affects the oral and dental health. Any chronic illness or deteriorating health issues will significantly undermine oral health. Any deterioration of oral health in turn contributes to decline of general health. Specific examples include the proven connection between gum disease (chronic low grade infection) and heart disease, hardening of the arteries and stroke. Diabetes also promotes gum disease through candida overgrowth (thrush) and acidosis (low pH). Low pH uses more calcium and magnesium to buffer acidosis making these essential minerals less available for the necessary continuous remineralization of teeth. This mineral imbalance contributes to the loss of enamel and the development of cavities because the saliva, which normally contains the building blocks of tooth enamel, becomes deficient in calcium and phosphate.

Any low grade chronic infection of the gums can travel through the blood stream to other organs and systems causing chronic illness and contributing to cognitive decline. Needed dental work for misalignment of teeth, for missing teeth and damaged teeth can contribute to attention disorders and cognitive weakness due to structural misalignment of the head and plates of the skull, the jaw, the neck and the spine which impair the optimal functions of the brain and nervous system. Good oral dental health also influences the self image and self esteem. Having needed dental work completed increases optimism and confidence and motivates improved hygiene and lifestyle choices to preserve that healthy smile.

Problems: Cracked teeth, braces, missing teeth, implants and bridges, injured teeth, cavities, broken teeth, loss of enamel

Root canals - decay close to a nerve causes inflammation, swelling and excruciating pain. Root canal drills out the nerve and leaves the now dead tooth in place and fills it or crowns it.

Crowns - replaces the top of a damaged tooth.

Implants - an 8mm long titanium or zirconium pin placed into the jaw as an anchor upon which to attach a screw on replacement tooth.

Whiteners - over bleaching causes burning gums and erosion of tooth enamel. Baking soda is an effective whitener.

Bad breath - has many causes, many of them bacterial. Poor hygiene and gum disease are the leading causes of bad breath. Tobacco, alcohol and sinus infection are all contributing factors. Additionally, poor digestion, liver disease, diabetes and cancer also promote bad breath. Probiotics and greens help to balance and detox the body.

GSE - grapefruit seed extract in water to fight infection and more frequent visits to the dental hygienist for professional cleaning is recommended. Three types of professional cleaning are available. The usual procedure for routine dental cleaning is scaling, scraping the teeth above and slightly below the gum line to remove plaque which causes tooth decay and gum disease. A second type of dental cleaning is called root planing. This is a deeper procedure that scrapes the degraded surface of the tooth down to smooth the surface and reduce gum irritation. There is also an oral irrigation procedure to flush below the gum line and kill germs. Older mouths need more frequent professional dental cleanings. Anyone who is having any dental problems should increase to three dental cleanings a year until their oral health has stabilized. After age 50, most people are benefited by an increase to three dental hygienists visits annually. It slows age related decline of oral health, cognitive health, heart health and immune health.

Failure to maintain oral health, including all needed repairs, can add ten years to the appearance of aging in the face; but even more significantly, it makes an even greater impact on the self concept as relates to aging, weakening, failing and feeling unattractive and undesirable. The use of veneers to cover damaged enamel and improve spacing contributes to improved health for the damaged but repaired teeth and improved psychological health for the self image as well.

Fluoride - okay, why fluoride? Coating the teeth with a fluoride solution promotes remineralization. Extra high doses of fluoride are what makes tooth paste for extra sensitive teeth work. It promotes remineralization of the enamel surfaces, reducing the nerve exposure and reducing sensitivity to hot and cold. However, excess of fluoride is toxic and results in loss of bone health due to fluoridosis.

Xylitol - the newer, safer way to remineralize teeth, is calcium glycerophosphate also called xylitol. It is available in many products that read positive +3.3 for oral dental health including Spry gum, Spry tooth gel and Spry mouth wash. For xylitol to have a beneficial effect, it needs to coat the tooth surfaces. Using it to cook with is not beneficial.

Toothpaste choices - the best precaution is to avoid sodium lauryl sulfate. Find something natural that you like or make your own tooth powder from xylitol and baking soda. Brush teeth until they really feel clean and smooth, not just till they taste clean. Yes, you really do have to clean in between the teeth. That can be done with floss, with a water pick or with tiny interdental brushes. This disruption of the plaque colonies must be done about every twenty four hours to prevent gingivitis, cavities and ultimately periodontal disease and tooth loss.

Toothbrush choices - it is best to have several and to use different ones, frequently changing from one to another, both manual and powered. If you like your toothbrush, you use it longer and more often. Depending on how many toothbrushes you are actively using, change them out for new ones every two to three months and after every acute illness, cold, fever, flu or vomiting. Always choose soft bristles so that vigorous brushing will not abrade the gums, leaving them more vulnerable to infection.

Fillings - choose ceramic, porcelain or resin composite. All three options read as zero, neutral, safe. Mercury amalgams read -3.6 which means it is not recommended because mercury is a dangerous neurotoxin and these fillings are outgassing a mercury vapor near the brain for about ten years after initial placement. This form of mercury is not as dangerous as the highly toxic methyl-mercury that is found in predatory fish but it is still a danger nonetheless. Removal of mercury fillings is usually the largest mercury toxin exposure event in a lifetime and should be done with great care and expertise, if at all.

Implants - the use of tiny titanium or zirconium pins, usually 8mm in length, set into the jaw bone. The pin serves as an anchor to hold an external post that screws into the implant. The external post holds the replacement tooth designed to fit that space exactly. Replacing a dead or missing tooth with a high quality implant can raise the oral dental health reading by as much as 3 points.

Gingivitis - red, swollen gums, bleeding when brushing teeth. Can be due to poor hygiene, malnutrition, thrush (a yeast overgrowth common with diabetes), cancer and the use of antibiotics. Causes bad breath.

Periodontal disease - a chronic acute gum disease characterized as more severe than gingivitis because this infection can travel through the blood stream to other organs and systems causing chronic illness including heart disease, hardening of the arteries, stroke and significant bone loss in the jaw and tooth loss. It is also associated with significant cognitive decline and immune system challenge.

Poor diet, acidosis and malnutrition weaken the jaw bone, the teeth and the immune system, causing tooth decay, gum disease and bone loss. Increased risk factors for oral dental health include hormone changes, stress, smoking, diabetes, alcoholism, drug addiction and STD's. Poor oral health significantly accelerates aging and cognitive decline. The proven solutions for oral health are hygiene, diet, hydration, pH and exercise as well as always getting repairs and reconstructions as needed. Watercress, wheatgrass, spinach and cilantro are especially beneficial for improving oral health.

Tooth infection can be addressed several ways:

GSE - grapefruit seed extract in water several times a day to coat the teeth and gums.
Oregano Oil Capsules - to fight infection in the deep tooth through improving antibiotic functions of the blood.
Vitamin C - Topical application of vitamin C powder directly onto inflamed or swollen gums.
Oral Vitamin C - 3 x a day, 2 grams per dose
Calcium, magnesium
Oil pulling - an Ayurvedic technique of swishing healthy oil in the mouth for a couple of minutes pulling it between the teeth. I have been asked to check on its benefits in a number of readings, but never has it been recommended as beneficial for any client. My impression is that it is simply inadequate to meet the challenges of any significant dental health issues.

CANCER

Cancer is a wound that doesn't heal. Whether on the skin or in the deeper organs, cancer is a failure of the body to repair damage and restore health. Cancer is always a state which is general to the whole body and all its systems. Cancer is never limited to local expression only at the site of its discovery. The general state of the body manifesting cancer is one of chronic over intoxication of the body's tissues due to weakness of liver and pancreatic functions. Over time this produces metabolic disturbance of the physiology of the whole organism at all levels; micro to macro, individual cellular biochemistry as well as organ and systems failures. Any combination of environmental, chemical, nutritional and genetic factors that produce a state of low pH in the kidneys and interstitial fluids (between cells) together with the chronic subclinical dehydration that accompanies acidosis (as well as produces it) will assuredly produce cancer of some type in less than 10 years.

About 80% of all diagnosed cancers appear to be clearly linked to environmental toxins which cause damage to the DNA of human cells which, if the cell doesn't die, produce cancerous mutations such that the cells continue to replicate but without the ability to repair damage. Thus the replicating cells are diseased, abnormal and producing systemic disease in the body. Cancerous tissue does not contain lymph vessels and normal repair of damaged cells is absent altogether.

Among the primary known carcinogens (agents that produce cancer) of our time tobacco is a clear leader considered directly responsible for 30% of all cancer deaths. Alcohol and tobacco combined produce cancers of both the mouth and gut. Medications and drugs are common carcinogens, including the direct relationship between the use of steroids to suppress inflammatory response and the subsequent development of liver cancer. Immunosuppressive drugs such as used for organ transplant as well as chemotherapy itself are well known for producing additional cancers. Chemical exposure through agriculture and industry, fertilizers, pesticides, dioxins and even the continuous exposure to estrogen mimicking polymers in petrochemical plastics have increased the cancer rates exponentially over the last 50 years.

Diet and specific food additives (such as the link between artificial sweeteners and bladder cancer) are well known for their carcinogenic effects. Radiation of all kinds is also know to damage cells without killing them, which is a primary cause of cancer. Asbestos produces cancer through microfiber cell damage and chronic inflammation. Electromagnetic radiation from high tension power lines or microwaves and cell phones are also cancer promoters in the segment of the population most vulnerable to electromagnetic challenge and the number of people affected is growing.

Viruses, called oncogenic viruses because they are known to produce cancer, include HPV, Hepatitis B and C, Epstein Barr (Mononeucleosis), Herpes and HIV. Bacteria are also know to produce cancers of the lungs as well as helicobacter pylori which can cause cancer in the gut. The least common causes of cancer are the known genetic predispositions such as BRCA1 and BRCA2 and defects of tumor suppressor gene p53.

The medical definition of cancer rests upon four different aspects which together indicate malignancy. First is the failure of normal cell development to progress to its end or terminal state called differentiation. Failure of cells to differentiate to their mature final function and form is abnormal cell development. These unhealthy cells that fail to mature into their normal function and form may have the potential to invade normal tissue and replace normal tissue with tissue forming from damaged DNA that does not have lymphatic cells and can not support the normal physiological process of healing at the level of the cell. The potential for the abnormal tissue growth to invade healthy tissue is the second criteria of malignancy. The third criteria is the potential for metastasis, the movement of the cells replicating with damaged DNA, through the lymph systems and blood vessels and establishing secondary sites of invading malignancy which may increase the danger to more critical organs. The fourth factor is called lethality.

Metastasizing cancer is more lethal. Cancer is cell synthesis from bad DNA that can repair its own telomeres and thus remain alive indefinitely and that can attract it's own blood supply to feed the abnormal tissue but that does not contain any lymph vessels and is thus deprived of the lymphatic function of detoxing the interstitial fluids between the cells to repair the cell damage. Thus the cancerous tissue is growing on its outer edges but dying and necrotic at its core. Cancer cells do not respond to normal metabolic signaling that tells irreparably damaged cells to self destruct. Instead these damaged cells keep replicating but cannot repair themselves. Where a cancer starts, in what kind of cells, determines what kind of cancer it is, no matter where it is found in the body.

Cancer Staging

Cancer staging is based on tumor size, involvement of local regional lymph nodes and distant metastasis.

Stage 1

Stage 1 cancer refers to a size of less than 2 cm, which is less than 1 inch and may be very much smaller. This designation of stage 1 also defines it as local to the primary diagnosed site with no appearance of cancer cells in the nearest lymph nodes and no distant metastasis. DCIS (ductal carcinoma in situ) is stage 1 cancer.

Stage 2

Stage 2 means the presence of the malignant cells in regional lymph nodes near the tumor.

Stage 3

Stage 3 indicates increasing size of malignancy with regional metastasis to lymph nodes but no proven distant metastasis - though they may be there.

Stage 4

Stage 4 cancer means all of the above and metastasis to distant organs and systems with ever increasing lethality. Tumors become more aggressive over time.

There are oncogenic promoter cells which can cause out of control growth factors in rapidly replicating cells. Estrogen and estrogen mimicking elements accelerate cell replication in malignant tissues. There are also tumor suppressor genes intended to stop the replication of damaged cells. Tumor suppressor gene p53 finds and repairs damaged cells or eliminates those that cannot be repaired. This gene is damaged or mutated in 50% of all cancers and 70% of colorectal cancers. Steroids are specifically known for reducing the body's natural tumor suppressing ability. Failures in the cellular metabolism to repair cell damage are promoted by acid pH of 6.4 and below. Lymphatic and vascular invasion of the malignant growth is accelerated by acid pH of 6.2 and below. Raising the pH of the body's interstitial fluids to 6.7 provides increased protection from the metabolic failures that produce cancer.

Medically, the malignant process, called carcinogenesis, begins with damage to normal cells which are injured but not killed, and which then mutate and replicate more abnormal cells. This is called activation and refers to an initiating event or exposure. Next comes the promotion of the abnormal cell metabolism by promoters which speed up or increase the replication of errors with mutations. Common promoters include the chemicals dioxin and DDT, artificial sweeteners saccharin and aspartame, cigarette smoke and aflatoxins from stored grain which promote liver cancer. Acidosis and dehydration are also promoters.

After activation and promotion, the stage referred to as conversion begins, when the malignancy is replicating abnormal cells that invade, metastasize and become lethal. All of this leads to the stage called progression, when the invasion and spread of cancer becomes clinically diagnosable disease, though the hidden disease has now existed for some time already. Conversion and progression are pH dependent aspects of this malignant process and are greatly accelerated by acidic pH of 6.2 and below in the interstitial fluids which is where the action of the lymph takes place to restore normal physiology.

A state of acidosis (low pH), dehydration, and increasing toxic burden retained in the cells is the ideal internal environment to support the development of any existing predisposition for cancer, and all predisposition to cancer, whether genetic, chemical or other damage, is infinitely more likely to manifest its worst potentials in this chronic state of deep disturbance and variance of vital metabolic functions outside of the range of normal human physiology. Restoring normal pH and hydration is essential to normal cell metabolism and is therefore essential to healing all chronic disease, no matter what the cause.

Healing Cancer is about transforming its meaning in your life. It is about healing hate and especially those things that we are proud to hate. Cancers most often appear in areas that represent what we hate in ourselves.

Causes:

Radiation (kidney cancer),
Chemicals (breast, brain and bone cancers),
Viruses (colon, ovarian, uterine, cervical HPV, lymphatic cancers)
Bacteria (prostate, helicobacter pylori and lung cancer)
Toxic Overload including smoking
Sunburn - skin cancer
Dehydration (prostate and bone cancers)
Suppressed diseases - gonorrhea, herpes, psoriasis
Genetic - damage to DNA
Repressed emotions, history of abuse and trauma

Treatments:

HYDRATION - 14 cups of water per day with Rescue Remedy, use structured water
ENEMAS - Flax oil, herb infusion, sea salt and baking soda - once every 10 days
EXERCISE - 50 minutes (or more) 5 days a week (or more)
Edgar Cayce Castor Oil packs once every 3 days for 30 repetitions of 3 hours each
DIET: Juice fasting - 4 to 6 ounces 4 x per day.
Raw juice 3 to 5 cups daily - to raise pH
Vegetarian diet (5% meat as broth) restrict animal fats, no whole meats, bone broth 3 cups broth daily
Elimination Diet - No refined grains, no GMO, HFCS, chocolate, canola, wheat, soy (to change the pH)
Organic, fresh, whole foods.
Eliminate processed, refined foods.
Use low sugar, less than 10%
Personal Spiritual Retreat - develops spiritual and emotional resilience
Journaling, emotional processing - supports self-realization
Massage: Neuromuscular, Reflexology, Lymphatic drainage

Supplements:

Vitamin C - oral 3 grams 3 x per day.
I.V. Vitamin C - 50 grams every 14 days or 25 grams every 7 days
Calcium disodium EDTA - 2 x day 1 gram per dose
CoQ10 - 300 mgs 2 x day
Quercetin - 4 grams 2 to 3 x day
Enzymes - digestive enzymes and food enzymes
Omegas - 2 grams per dose 2 x day
Wheat grass juice, barley green - live green juice (spinach, watercress) is better than any processed powder Green Vibrance
Acidophilus, Ruteri
Floradix Epresat vitamin formula and liquid magnesium formula
Vitamin B100 complex - 2 x day and Folic Acid 800 mcgs

Botanicals:

GSE - grapefruit seed extract, antibiotic, antiviral immune support
Oregano oil
Reishi mushrooms - lymphatic support, stimulates macrophages

Mistletoe, toxic herb, useful only under the guidance of a trained professional
Chaparral, a toxic herb, useful for detox enemas
Burdock, Slippery Elm, Red Clover (Essiac) and Kelp Flor-Essence)
Cordyceps Mushrooms - stimulates production of interferon
Maitake mushrooms - stimulates production of interluekin-1 and boosts energy
Beets, water cress, wheatgrass juice
Amazon Herbs - Envirozon, Recovazon and Shipibo Treasure Tea

HEALTHY SKIN

Sugar causes wrinkles. Alcohol causes wrinkles. Smoking causes wrinkles. Sun causes wrinkles and aging causes wrinkles. Liver weakness causes rashes and sores. Kidney weakness also causes rashes and sores and split nails. Both also cause heel cracks.

Healthy skin depends on healthy organs and systems, healthy nutrition and hormone levels as well as lifestyle choices that protect skin from external dangers of toxic exposures and injuries. Healthy skin reflects overall general health and unhealthy skin indicates the inner challenge in the manifestation on the skin. Because the skin is visible, it is often the motivation for addressing the deeper problem. Skin problems effect self esteem and social standing. It is important to look good and feel good in our own skin. It is our first costume, our birthday suit. The skin gives early warning signs of deeper weakness that could otherwise go long undetected, undiagnosed or underestimated.

Eczema is usually an indication of kidney weakness and is often associated with asthma in the weakest constitutions. Psoriasis is a different type of skin lesion that is produced by liver weakness leading to the body's over dependance on detoxing through the skin to eliminate toxins that would normally have been processed through the liver and colon. Hormone imbalances cause both acne and severe dry skin. Food allergies, chemical allergies and pet allergies can produce rashes, hives and welts.

Keeping the body pure of those things which cause damage will produce a younger healthier looking skin. By the time you are old enough to really care just how much younger you will look without all those exposures, it is much too late. Avoiding all the negatives will make skin look ten to twenty years younger fifty years down the road. Look around and you will see that many people choose to experience all that life has to offer and accept the wrinkles that come with those choices, reserving the right to make surgical and laser treatment choices at a later date if they can afford it. Others choose to avoid all the pitfalls and protect their skin from aging by constant vigilance. Those who make their living from their looks are the most careful and invest the most time and money in skin care. But then all of us are affected in our income to some degree by how we look, not just models and actresses. The better looking person often gets more easily hired for the better job. The better looking person gets treated better by co-workers and colleagues. The better looking person invests more time and concern in the self care of getting real needs met. Everyone has different ideas about what constitutes better looking but we all agree that it includes healthy skin.

A symptom on the surface of the skin is a message from the body about its internal state of affairs. When pursuing constitutional healing, the direction of cure includes the movement of disease from deeper more critical organs to the skin. This produces rashes and lesions that are expressions of the disease moving out of the body. They can persist for weeks, for months or even for years, depending on the magnitude of the challenge being relieved. Careful attention to the nature of and changes in any rashes, boils, hives, ulcerations and skin lesions of any kind is always important.

Some chronic diseases cause skin itching, irritation and rashes, including diabetes, cancer and candida. They also contribute to poor wound healing. Hormone balance, essential fatty acid balance, nutritional deficiencies, dehydration and poor elimination of toxins due to kidney or liver weakness will all show in the quality of the skin. Persistent nail fungus is a sign of deeper fungal infection in the kidneys that will not resolve by applications to the nails alone. Support for clearing the fungal infection from the deeper organs will help heal toe and finger nail fungus.

Skin plays a significant role in the regulation of body temperature. The pores of the skin close to retain heat and they open to release heat. The skin cools the body even more rapidly when wet with sweat. Unhealthy skin, scars over 65% of the body, which can happen from burns or psoriasis, is enough to disrupt the normal body temperature control mechanisms. The ability to then rely on regulations of the temperature of the environment can become crucial because the body cannot readily adapt to either heat or cold.

To support healthy skin, hair and nails use a bone marrow broth 2 to 3 cups daily for three or four months. Raw juice and raw food are also important because they provide the increased plant sourced progesterone, the skin hormone. Even more important than these nutritional contributions to healthy skin is continuous super hydration with structured water. For topical support, use aloe vera gel, jojoba oil, carrot seed oil and calendula ointments. Do not use products that contain Sodium Laurel Sulfate, Triclosan, Phthalates, Parabens, ammonia and formaldehyde.

Allergic:

Hives, wheals, welts - red, raised, water filled, itchy.

Causes:

Antibiotics and other medications, nuts, shellfish and food allergies, insects. Treatments: ice, Quercitin, Rescue Remedy, Oral EDTA, Arsenicum or other homeopathics

Contact Dermatitis

Causes: chemicals, solvents, detergents, cosmetics, jewelry, fabric, or plants. For poison ivy/oak use Jewelweed (Oak away), Quercitin, Aloe Vera gel, Rhus Tox

Non-Infectious Heat Rash

Heat rash/prickly heat - sweaty areas, itches and burns. Keep cool and dry, apply ice or cold mint poultice. Cornstarch.

Boils

Boils raised, pus filled red bump. Vitamin C, Pycnogenols, Cordyceps, hot poultices. Usually caused by Staphylococcus or remedy aggravation. GSE

Eczema

Eczema - dry, red, itchy, possibly wet, weepy. Cause - usually kidney weakness, wheat, nitrites. Topical MSM, Calendula. Pulsatilla, Silica, Sulphur or Petroleum

Psoriasis

Psoriasis - pink, raised, flaky, crusty, scales, may bleed. Usually liver weakness, toxic overload and stress. Quercetin, Alpha Lipoic Acid, CoQ10, Prid ointment, pycnogenols, burdock, carrot seed oil, epsom salts baths, castor oil packs, energy work. Staphysagria

Rosacea

Rosacea, redness of the skin over the nose and cheeks, rough rashy look, irritated skin, itchy bumps that go through cycles of improvement and reoccurrence. Liver, toxic overload. Causes include alcohol and dehydration. Rosacea is a sign of deep constitutional disturbance involving liver weakness and specific triggers producing inflammation. Known triggers include alcohol, high sugar / high insulin levels and becoming overheated or overstressed. Determining specific triggers and eliminating them is usually essential. Alcohol and sun exposure are the most common triggers of acute flare ups, but for many others, food allergens must be avoided. Hydrogenated oils, rancid oils and cooked oils (as in fried foods) all aggravate the condition because the weakened liver is unable to metabolize these fats and elimination of toxins from the blood is impaired. Healing the digestive system, the liver, the immune system and allergies, are all part of recovery from rosacea. Alpha lipoic acid and digestive enzymes are frequently beneficial. Exercise is also essential to restore liver health but caution to prevent over heating and exercise induced sweating is recommended. Homeopathics Pulsatilla and Sulphur 50M and CM potencies.

Treatments:

Elimination diet, ginger tea, Green Vibrance, lemon juice, castor oil packs. Sulphur, Pulsatilla, structured water, exercise.

Acne

Acne is usually diet, hormone balance and stress. Cordyceps, Burdock, Vitamin A, hypericum tincture, Myrrh.

Dry Skin

Paper thin, deep wrinkles, emollients do not relieve - hormone imbalance, use ProGest cream liberally. Calendula, aloe vera gel, carrot seed oil.

Candida

Yeast overgrowth - sugar imbalance. Green Vibrance, hydration, diet, GSE.

Infectious / Contagious

Impetigo

Bacterial strep infection, crusty, weeping, spreads. Myrrh. Staphysagria.

Chicken Pox

Virus, fever, cold symptoms, vesicles appear on trunk first, itchy, weepy. Oatmeal baths, calamine, fever reducer. Pulsatilla

Measles

Virus, fever, eyes sensitive, flat, diffuse pink rash. Contagious for 10 days after rash appears and 2 days before (same as Chicken Pox) Calamine, fever reducer, oatmeal baths, Sulphur, Pulsatilla, Rescue Remedy

Roseola

Virus, infants, high fever followed by diffuse rash. Contagious 4 days after rash appears and 2 days before. Sulphur

Ringworm

Tinea - fungal. Often from kittens. Micatin or Tinactin, Taraxacum, iron deficiency.

Cancers Melanoma

10% of all skin cancers. Mole, birthmark, changes in size or shape, irregular border. Kidneys. Sanguinaria, black salve, goldenseal, I.V. vitamin C

Basal Cell Carcinoma

75% of all skin cancers, slowest form, a sore that doesn't heal, crusts and bleeds. Liver disease. Green Vibrance, CoQ10, Zinc, lemon juice, Salt scrubs, castor oil pack over liver and omentum, general detoxing, Vitamin C, Vespera Serum.

Squamous Cell Carcinoma

More aggressive, tends to spread, hard, scaly, crusty, appears on lips, ears, hands, neck and arms. Environmental toxins, diet and emotional health. I.V. Vitamin C or EDTA, Oral Vitamin C,

Cordyceps, Essiac, Chaparral, Kombuchu, castor oil packs, epsom salts baths, Acetyl L-carnitine, Rescue Remedy, Vespera Serum.

Treatments:
Castor oil packs poultices
Epsom salts baths
Elimination diet - peanuts, wheat, shellfish, pork, citrus, melons, food additives and colorings, sulfites, nitrites, alcohol, prescription and nonprescription medications
Eat Organic only
Energy work for healing the psyche

Topicals:

Calendula, Prid ointment, hypericum tincture, carrot seed oil, Myrrh, MSM, tea tree oil, jewelweed - Oak Away, mint, ice, cornstarch, ProGest cream, Micatin or Tinactin anti-fungal cream, aloe vera gel, Calamine, Black Salve, Vespera Serum, hydrogen peroxide in the bath water, epsom salts baths, sea salt baths

Supplements And Botanicals:

EDTA for chelating out toxins, orally, I.V. or in the bath water
Vitamin C - oral and I.V.
Quercetin - for allergic outbreaks or hyperimmune symptoms
Vitamin A
Vitamin E
Iron
Zinc
MSM - dissolved in water, apply topically
Structured Water
CoQ10
GSE - antibiotic, antiviral, anti-fungal
Essiac
Burdock
Chaparral
Goldenseal
Sanguinaria
Cordyceps mushrooms
Omega's
Green Vibrance, watercress, wheatgrass juice - for liver cleanse

Lemon juice in water 8 x day for kidney cleanse
Rescue Remedy topically and orally
Carrot Seed Oil, topically (dilute in jojoba oil)
ProGest Cream - progesterone is the skin hormone

Skin lesions can cause severe suffering and relief is a high priority. Epsom salt baths is a first line of defense. The body readily absorbs the magnesium dissolved in the water through the skin. It promotes shedding of dead tissue and is soothing.

Sea salt baths are also helpful but may sting open sores. A combination of both epsom salts and sea salt (a cup or more of each) is another choice for relieving itch and pain and reducing redness, inflammation and infection. Hydrogen peroxide in the bath water also fights infection and speeds healing. Use 1 cup in a standard size bath. For severe outbreaks on the skin which are not resolving, I.V. vitamin C often will provide rapid relief and speed up recovery.

Because these skin lesions are active sores coming from within, they often itch, sting, burn or otherwise drive the sufferer to utter distraction. Scratching and picking at these sores is pretty normal, however, finger nails are dirty and may introduce a secondary infection. Clothing, bedding and other surfaces can also introduce infection into open wounds. In this case, sores become bright red, inflamed, swollen and may itch and sting. Topical application of a triple antibiotic ointment (such as Neosporin) three times a day will fight infection as well as soften the distressed skin and reduce breaks in the friable tissue. If secondary infection is not a concern then calendula ointment can be used instead.

If there is any concern that a skin lesion may be melanoma, do not wait to get it checked by a professional. Melanoma is common, can advance rapidly and is very dangerous when it does. For lesions that are not cancer, topical application of Vespera Serum (by Exuvience) can speed up cell renewal and skin regeneration. It also clears scars and stretch marks.

Herpes / Shingles

Herpes is a virus that remains in the body between outbreaks, lying dormant in the nerves of the spine. It re-emerges whenever there is an immune system collapse due to trauma, injury, chronic and acute illness, surgery and chemotherapy. Shingles is due to a re-emergence of the virus varicella zoster which causes chicken pox. One out of every three people who have had chicken pox will experience an acute episode of shingles when the immune system is compromised due to severe illness, cancer, chemotherapy, organ or stem cell transplant, immunosuppressive drugs, shock and trauma. There are one million new cases of shingles each year in the U.S. Recovery can take 6 months or longer.

Symptoms: blister clusters with pain, tingling, fever, malaise.
Oral Herpes -Emotion - SHAME. Resides in the cervical spine. Recovery time 10 days.
Genital Herpes - Emotion - NOT GOOD ENOUGH. Lumbar spine. Recovery 14 days.
Shingles - Emotion - COLLAPSE or WORTHLESS. Usually above the waist, 5-9 weeks acute phase often with pain lingering for several months. Shingles is common with radiation therapy.

Treatments:

Kneipp Valerian and Hops Bath
Topical MSM, calendula tincture and aloe vera gel
Ice and minted ice
Poultice of mint and comfrey (not hot)
Hydrogen peroxide, 1 cup in the bath water

Supplements And Botanicals:

Floradix - Floravital with Iron and Herbs - 3 x day or Epresat Green Vibrance
Acidophilus (mixed) - 3 x day
Quercetin - 4 grams 3 x day
Vitamin C - 2 grams 3 x per day, also I.V.
Vitamin C therapy
Ginger Tea - 6 cups daily (fresh), also lemon juice 3 x day
Vitamin B 100 complex - 2 x day
Lysine - 1,000 mgs 2 x day for 4 weeks, repeat for every outbreak
Structured Water - 2 to 3 liters daily
Rescue Remedy - 3 droppers full in Structured Water
GSE - grapefruit seed extract, 2 caps per dose 3 x day or 3 drops in water 4 x a day
Oregano Oil capsules - 3 x per day with meals
Ashwaganda - 2 capsules per day
Colostrum - 2 x day
Elderberry syrup - 3 x day in water
Energy work, cranio sacral adjustments, emotional release work
Acyclovir - Zovirax, safe topical gel
Homoepathic Arsenicum, Nat. Mur., Veratrum Alb., Zincum Phos. or Phosphorus
Stress management and relaxation
Lower activity level, realistic expectations

FIBROMYALGIA

Affects up to 10 million Americans, 85% of them women.

Until quite recently, Fibromyalgia was a mystery disease, difficult to diagnose and easily confused with or mistaken for Chronic Fatigue Syndrome, Rheumatoid Arthritis or Lyme's disease. Over the last three decades, a clear picture has finally emerged from the evidence and experience of over ten million patients. In the words of today's leading experts, fibromyalgia begins when the patient's body metaphorically 'blows a fuse'. A systems overload that results from an energy crisis of expending more energy than the body is capable of producing or maintaining. Fibromyalgia presents with wide spread pains all over the body that persists for months, often accompanied by insomnia and exhaustion. This combination of pain and weakness will often lead to depression if effective relief is not achieved.

Fibromyalgia always presents with dehydration due in part to nutritional crisis causing acidosis, but also due to over production of cortisol. Adrenal exhaustion or adrenal failure together with weak thyroid health are often accompanied by opportunistic infections including candida, as well as viral or bacterial infections due to the generally weakened and vulnerable state of immune functions which are suppressed when cortisol levels are high. Progesterone levels are low due to high cortisol and both hormonal anomalies contribute to sleeplessness.

Rebalancing hormones can be supported with progesterone cream, maca and stress management. Replacement of minerals including magnesium, calcium, potassium, iron, iodine and salt is essential to restoring fluid balance and pH. GSE can be used to fight any infections that may also be present.

Symptoms: Chronic generalized muscle pain, tenderness, stiffness, aching, weakness, fatigue, INSOMNIA, depression, weak concentration, headaches, allergic response to foods and environment.

Causes: Endocrine Failure - adrenal (insufficiency), thyroid, pituitary (overstimulation)

Leaky Gut Syndrome - sensitizes the body to wheat, dairy, tomato, potato, rancid oils Candida overgrowth promotes acidosis (and dehydration)
Dehydration - chronic subclinical dehydration, insufficient water intake

Spiritual/Emotional: Taking on too much including other's stuff, other's feelings and outlook, co-dependence, poor boundaries, failure to rest.

Treatments: Conventional allopathic medicine - None. Attempts to control symptoms with anti-depressants and anti-inflammatory medicines which cause further dehydration.

Natural Therapies:

EDTA - oral or I.V.
Fresh ginger Tea - 5 cups daily. Heals thyroid and leaky gut.
Super HYDRATE - 3 liters of Structured water daily
ProGest Cream - progesterone cream to support adrenals, thyroid, smooth muscles and circulation and promote sleep.
Colonics - every 14 days for 5 repetitions.
Edgar Cayce castor oil packs over the omentum, liver, and intestines every 3 days for 25 repetitions of 3 hours each.
Massage - lymphatic drainage and relaxation, every 7 days for 10 repetitions or more.
Exercise 60 minutes daily 6 days a week.
Raw Juice - 3 cups daily to raise pH
Emotional processing, journaling

Supplements And Botanicals:

Progesterone Cream
Flor-Essence liquid detox formula x 4 weeks
Wilson's Thyroid Px
Melatonin - 3 to 5 mgs
CoQ10 - 400 mgs 2 x daily
Omega's - 2 grams 2 x day, per dose –Vegans and Vegetarians use Flax oil 2,000 mgs 2 x day
Alpha Lipoic Acid - 600 mgs 2 x day.
Metabolic Maintenance
Vitamin B 100 complex once or twice a day
Quercetin - 3 grams per dose 3 x per day
Acidophilus - mixed, 3 x per day and 3 x the indicated dose
Enzymes - 3 x day. Source Naturals

Magnesium - by Natural Calm 500 mgs 2 x day

Adrenal glandular tissue tablets (or thyroid)

GSE - to fight infections increase protein to lower cortisol levels, broth, sprouts and raw nut creams

Vitamin C - oral and I.V. to heal adrenals

Maca Powder - raw, mix into raw juice, 2 to 3 tablespoons daily

Cordyceps Mushrooms - to detox lymph. 3 capsules per dose 2 x day.

Kneipp Lavender Bath - adrenal support, balancing. 3 to 5 times per week.

WOMENS SEXUAL AND REPRODUCTIVE HEALTH

There are three normal phases of female health. The prepubescent phase, non-menstruating and not physiologically prepared for sex - including physically, mentally and emotionally - all of which are regulated by hormone chemistry. The second phase lasts about thirty years wherein the body's hormones and physiology support the development of an active sex life, including menstruation and the possibility of conception and birth. The third phase is non-menstruating, non fertile and sexual activity is less driven by hormones and determined more by deeper considerations. The needs of the individual differ vastly from one stage to the next.

In phase one, a young girl needs to learn how to keep herself clean and dry. She also can learn to use a calendula ointment on her genitals if they are slightly or mildly irritated. Some young girls have yeast overgrowth called candida that causes a discharge, inflammation, tenderness and cracking of delicate tissues and intense red skin. A candida diet that restricts processed foods and sugar will be needed to restore balance. Grapefruit seed extract inhibits yeast overgrowth quite effectively but it tastes bad. When using drops, put about 4 drops into an ounce of water and repeat the dose three or four times a day. It is also available in capsules. Increase the probiotic reuteri which fights yeast and, for girls over the age six consider an over the counter candida cleanse formula at the natural market if the problem is not fully controlled by the elimination diet together with the probiotic and GSE.

A child's sexual identity is pretty well established in her self image by age three, though it is still highly malleable until age seven. Gender orientation is largely based in three factors: hormone chemistry, social conditioning (especially parental preferences when punishing for behaviors) and thirdly, the environmental chemistry including exposures through food, water, air and medications that are hormone disrupters. Heterosexual, homosexual or bisexual orientations do not read as good, bad, right or wrong in the attunements. They are just a personal and cultural format for giving expression to the self concept.

Girls need to know about the menstrual cycle by age six and need more complete information about how that will effect them by age 11. They will need education about sexually transmitted diseases and birth control by age 14. A young girl and her family also face a difficult decision about the highly controversial vaccine meant to reduce the risk of cervical cancer due to human papilloma virus.

The vaccine is controversial because thousands of young women claim to have been seriously injured by it, some within 48 hours after the first injection and many almost immediately after the second dose. The vaccine is given as a series of 3 shots. These injured girls have posted videos of themselves before and after their immunizations to document the real life outcome from their own firsthand experience. In tens of thousands of cases, the outcome may be absolutely tragic.

Healthy Birth Control

Most sexually active people need to consider birth control options and there are now more choices than ever: the pill, the sponge, the IUD, the ring, the patch, the shot, the implant, the diaphragm, condoms and ovulation awareness through cervical mucus.

Only the last three methods listed can be considered natural. Ovulation awareness works well when combined with the use of condoms or diaphragm, but is usually recommended only for couples who are planning a family and for whom a pregnancy would not be an unacceptable disaster. The diaphragm itself, which is a barrier to conception, is natural, but the spermicide used with it is not and will cause a reaction in sensitive individuals. The cervical cap functions also as a barrier and is used with spermicide, however it has proven less adaptable to the cervix that has given birth and therefore less reliable as birth control for those who have already had a child. The spermicidal sponge is also considered less effective for those who have already given birth because it is less likely to stay in the most effective position over the cervix. The sponge is also very messy and may drip for hours. There is one more significantly effective non-hormonal contraceptive, the copper IUD. The copper IUD is safer than the plastic IUD that releases hormones. IUD's are considered a high risk factor for pelvic inflammatory disease because they may facilitate the movement of chlamydia and gonorrhea into the deeper organs, including the uterus and fallopian tubes.

Many forms of hormonal birth control are now available by prescription, including dozens of different pills, a patch, a shot that lasts for three months, the plastic implant that goes in the arm, the ring that releases hormones into the vagina for three weeks every month and then gets replaced, and the plastic hormone releasing IUD.

All forms of hormone-based contraception are considered more dangerous for cigarette smokers. Other risks associated with hormonal contraception include bleeding and blood clot disorders, increased risk of cancer and risk of long term hormone imbalance, particularly after the three month shot.

Diabetes, heart disease, family history of breast or reproductive cancer, high blood pressure, stroke and nursing a baby are all contra-indications for the use of hormone based birth control. The new birth control pill designed to limit menstruation to only four cycles per year is the most dangerous form of hormonal birth control available today and can produce bleeding anomalies that may remain when the prescription is discontinued, and in some cases, it results in continued infertility.

Safely protecting oneself from both STD's and unwanted pregnancies takes responsibility, knowledge and consciousness. Recovering from not successfully protecting oneself from these challenges will alter the course of many lives. In the U.S. over nineteen million patients are diagnosed with new STD's every year and another fifteen million new cases are going undiagnosed each year.

Fibroids

Perhaps half of all adult women will have uterine fibroids at some point, though a majority of them may never be aware of these non-cancerous tumors growing out of uterine tissue. Liver health, including efficiency of filtering toxins from the blood and the estrogen balance, particularly when disrupted by estrogen mimicking polymers in plastics, chemicals and prescription drugs, is a primary source of these growths of abnormal tissue. Diagnosis is made by ultrasound. Minimally invasive fibroid removal called myomectomy, which leaves the uterus intact, is the usual course of treatment if the fibroids cause symptomatic problems such as heavy bleeding and back pain. Hormones are often given to shrink the tumors before this surgery. If the underlying constitutional health remains unchanged, fibroids are likely to recur. The best treatment is improved diet, physical fitness and stress reduction. Hormone replacement therapy can promote fibroid growth.

Preconception, Pregnancy, Birth and Recovery

Almost half of all pregnancies in the U.S. carried to term (not aborted or miscarried) are planned. Sometimes it is because conception didn't just happen that a couple begins to look into conscious preparation for conception. All those choices which support health in general are necessary to the fullest degree to support healthy pregnancy. Physical fitness does not improve significantly after conception and is of particular importance for supporting the mother through the rigors of labor and delivery. Greater physical fitness means a healthier baby, a shorter labor, an easier delivery, and a speedier recovery after birth. Lack of physical fitness contributes to dysfunctional labor and delayed recovery for the mother. Because the mother's body is flooded with HCG, the hormone that allows the placenta to implant in the uterine wall, she will likely experience nausea and vomiting and unusually low energy for the first three months of pregnancy. This challenge of the pregnancy itself stands in the way of all good intentions to maintain or increase physical fitness.

By the time this stage of feeling generally unwell and exhausted has passed, the pregnancy is well advanced and increasing physical fitness remains difficult.

Equal in importance is preconception nutrition for both parents. Increasing vitamin B complex and folic acid together with a supplement of omega's provides protection from neural tube defects like Spinabifida and builds strong healthy brains and nervous systems. This may be beneficial for the prevention of autism and improved development of cognitive intelligences. Preventing toxemia of pregnancy and gestational diabetes both are accomplished only by eating a diet that meets the needs of the mother's body to produce a fifty percent increased blood supply. That is one hundred and fifty percent of the blood volume of a non-pregnant woman. Not only does that require super nutrition, the baby's liver is storing iron and building a body, which also requires lots of protein.

A high sugar, high starch diet, such as is common in America, leads to weakness of the muscles due to high insulin levels. This weakness prolongs labor, makes it inefficient and leads to complications of birth including the increased need for pitocin and likelihood of postpartum hemorrhage.

Strength through nutrition and exercise must be further supported by sleep, rest and lower stress levels to keep the expectant mother from becoming depleted physically and over extended emotionally. Trying to keep up the pre-pregnant pace of expectations, both for work and socially, is not ideal. Taking time out for pregnancy, however, has become a privilege that is not available to all. Some situations do not allow the mother to take off personal time before the birth and often require the mother to return to work before she can fully recover. The higher the stress level and the activity level in general, the greater the increase in the body's need for extra sleep and extra rest. Those are two separate things. Time to get off her feet repeatedly throughout the day is as important as exercise when it comes to preserving strength and stamina.

For labor and delivery, it is best to have a doula in addition to your labor and delivery team. The doula is trained in guiding the mother and supporting the mother through birth. This is like having a personal assistant looking out for you, in addition to your doctors and nurses. The doula may be able to help you better create the birth experience you want to have or to better cope with the one you are having. She can help you be better informed about choices and options, about what is going on, and provide more emotional support than may otherwise be available. Kudos to the doulas for their much needed expertise and the improved birth experiences they support.

Before the birth, parents need to make a decision about vaccination at birth. If they wish to delay immunization, they will need to discuss that with their doctor. Families that have experienced several generations of special needs brains such as autism, seizure disorders, bi-polar disorder and mental illness, will be more likely to research vaccines extensively and make choices that consider their specific vulnerabilities of brain and nervous system.

I do not recommend that either mother or baby receive any immunizations immediately after birth. I advocate for a well considered delay while the infant immune system comes to maturity and is more resilient in the face of the challenge. I also advocate for fewer immunizations total and that those vaccines are carefully and specifically chosen for each child or each person. However, the model I have just advocated for is not the prevailing model advocated by big medicine and it is not a choice that is fully supported by law in some states. People who believe in vaccines should not be empowered to force them on people who do not share their beliefs. If this were the case, the quality of vaccines available would greatly improve because they would have to satisfy market demand for highest quality and safety to sell their product.

Recovery from birth is perhaps one of the most overlooked and taken for granted aspects of health today. The challenge to the mother's body is minimized both in her mind and in the outlook of those around her. Mothers are expected to do it all and have no real needs. We have a social or cultural fantasy that mothers will recuperate normally after birth and recover their strength even if the pregnancy became high risk, the birth complicated, and the mother did not have adequate help and resources.

The reality is that without careful attention to the mother's real needs for recovery, each succeeding child will be less healthy than those before. Spacing children farther apart, such as four to five years, greatly improves the mother's likelihood of restoring full vibrant health and passing it on to her children. The health of the mother determines the health of the baby.

Menopause

Menopause, also called change of life, is the end of the fertile phase of female development. The cessation of the menstrual cycle and ovulation is normal at about or just after age fifty, though early menopause can occur. Menopausal symptoms associated with this change can be indicators of other health risks including dehydration, acidosis, osteoporosis, circulatory weakness including heart disease and other hormonal weakness including adrenal and thyroid. Menopause has a way of drawing attention to the need to take responsibility for better self care including diet, exercise and stress management.

Being nutritionally challenged, emotionally distressed, and physically depleted increases the severity of hormone imbalance and the related hot flashes and the risk of depression. This is a time of re-assessment and rebuilding for the future. Failure to respond to this change of life phase with a corresponding change of lifestyle usually results in an inner adjustment of identity and self concept that accelerates aging both physically and in the personality, including loss of sexual desire.

Menopause can be a wake-up call to those who have always promised themselves that they would one day catch up on getting their real needs met.

Menopause, Change Of Life

Begins between the age of 45 and 55 years, in America average is 52 years.

Spiritual Emotional Issues:

The key word here is CHANGE and taking responsibility for creating change you want. Identity and self examination, the next grandest version of you.

Symptoms:

Hot flashes, night sweats, insomnia, low libido, vaginal dryness, slowed metabolism, hypothyroid, weight gain, dry skin and aging, anxiety and depression.

Causes:

Decreased hormone levels, especially progesterone due to loss of corpus luteum as source.
Adrenal Exhaustion, high stress, overwork (progesterone is further depleted if cortisol is high)
Poor Diet, over eating, caffeine, sugar, highly refined processed foods, alcohol, acidosis
sedentary lifestyle, lack of physical fitness, strength and stamina
Xenoestrogens - environmental toxins that bind with estrogen receptors including herbicides, pesticides, plastics, detergents, hormones and prescription medications in water supply and in food supply
Heavy Metals and Toxins - Mercury, Arsenic, Cadmium, Fluoride and glyphosate

Treatments:

Diet, proper hydration, prevention of acidosis
Eliminate alcohol for at least 4-6 months and then restrict to no more than 2 alcoholic drinks per month
Exercise 60 minutes per day 5 -7 days a week.
Walking, Yoga, Chi Gong or Tai Chi.
Progesterone Cream - ProGest, 1/2 teaspoon 2 x per day
Lower stress levels, practice balance and repose, lower activity levels meditation, processing, self examination and choice, journaling, prayer
Massage
Acupuncture - balance adrenals/hormones
Raw Juice - 2 to 3 cups daily for pH, hydration and progesterone source

Supplements And Botanicals:

ProGest Cream - twice a day, bone building hormone and fat metabolism, sleep hormone and skin hormone.

Flax Seed Oil - 3 times a day, 2 capsules per dose (vegetarian sourced omegas)

PhytoEstrogens - Gaia Herbs (vitex, cohosh, clover, sage and others) balances estrogen

CoQ10 - 200 mgs 2 x a day

Vitamin B complex - B-100's daily

Vitamin C - 2 grams per dose 3 x a day

Vitamin E - 400 I.U.'s 2 x a day

Omegas - 2 grams per dose 2 x a day

Maca Powder - 2 to 4 tablespoons per day, mixed into raw juice, raw pies and bliss balls

Acidophilus, particularly Reuteri - for production of vitamin K and vitamin D

Pregnenelone - precursor to all steroid hormones including progesterone and cortisol, adrenal support

Alpha lipoic acid - for brain, liver and circulatory health

HRT - synthetic estrogens and progestins have produced increased incidence of blood clots, asthma and liver and gallbladder weakness. Contraindicated with Cancer, clotting disorders, obesity and diabetes. Estrogen therapy is always for the shortest time possible. Less that two years is best.

Bio-Identical Hormones - non synthetic but also promotes estrogen dominance

Unopposed estrogen (not balanced by progesterone) predisposes to weight gain and water retention edema, increased clotting incidence, excretion of magnesium and zinc and the depletion of mineralization of bones including calcium

MENS HEALTH - SEXUAL AND REPRODUCTIVE

A man's sexual and reproductive health is interdependent upon his overall general health as well as specifically his heart health, both his physical heart and his emotional heart, his adrenal health, kidney health, thyroid health and his blood sugar. Keeping physically fit with regular exercise and eating a diet of unprocessed whole natural foods is the best support for healthy libido, healthy self image, healthy relationships and vigorous responsiveness of the sexual organs.

Reduced erectile function and responsiveness is a common challenge and the cause is rarely anything other than lifestyle choices and habits. High pressure, high stress personalities that indulge in angry outbursts to vent their frustrations and perhaps control those around them are prime candidates for ever increasing episodes of reduced erectile responsiveness. These same habits of anger and stress as an ongoing personality style are also known to contribute to the development of heart disease called atherosclerosis. The same hinderance of circulation that is occurring in the arteries supplying the heart are also occurring in the much smaller blood vessels supplying the flow that supports erection. High stress and high cortisol promote erectile dysfunction.

Mens sexual responsiveness is profoundly affected by alcohol because it uses up hydration, makes pH more acidic, and raises blood sugar and insulin levels, all of which reduce healthy blood flow to genitals. Alcohol also causes lower testosterone levels. A few drinks in the evening will still be affecting ability to perform for as much as 24 hours and can rob you of the anticipated next morning sex even with eight hours of sleep after last nights drinks.

It takes about three months of changed habits, lower sugar, less or no alcohol, increased exercise and improving metabolism to produce increased sexual vitality, sexual function and fertility. Additionally, specific herbs, nutrients and supplements have long been used and proven effective in increasing sexual vitality, stamina, performance and personal satisfaction. The amino acid L-arginine helps dilate blood vessels to support erectile response, however, the amount needed of 3 to 4 grams daily can disrupt the lysine balance of a man who has herpes. If herpes is part of the constitutional picture its usually best not to rely on L-arginine supplementation for support. Fish oil and Omega 3 supplementation along with co-enzyme CoQ10 in moderate to high amounts seems well indicated in almost all cases.

Two grams twice daily of Omegas and 300 to 400 mgs of CoQ10 - 2 x day will safely support heart health, circulation, brain functions and sexual functions. Nature has provided several options to choose from for food sourced erectile & hormone support. Watermelon increases nitric oxide levels and improves hydration which together provide significant support for erection. Maca powder, imported from Peru, provides food sourced hormone support that heals adrenal and liver functions as well as increasing stamina and vitality that improve performance and sexual satisfaction. Other herbs known for safe effective support of sexual health are tribulus terrestris, long jack, and a extract of fenugreek called testofen. A combination of these herbs can, in some cases, produce higher testosterone levels and an increased experience of sexual well being. The herb saw palmetto is also frequently recommended as a male supplement because it effectively reduces prostate enlargement. However, saw palmetto may also reduce fertility and therefore should only be used with a conscious awareness of both of these two potential actions. Many prescription medications, including those for high blood pressure, have pronounced side effects which affect hormone balance, kidney function and produce impotence or erectile disfunction. Healing the sexual functions will usually require healing the problem for which the medication is prescribed as well.

Impotence

Affects 30 million American men

Causes:

Medications, especially anti-depressants and blood pressure meds.
Alcohol, chronic acidosis and dehydration.
Circulatory disease, heart disease, diabetes, high cholesterol, low testosterone, low zinc, hypothyroid, hypopituitary, Parkinson's, MS
Anxiety, depression, guilt, shame, boredom
Poor physical fitness
Cancer and surgery (especially prostate surgery).

Natural Therapies:

Exercise 60 minutes a day - increases testosterone levels and core fitness
Maintain appropriate weight - especially around the belly

Maintain hydration (it takes +4 hydration to support erectile function)

Zinc - effects pituitary and hormone levels, 30 to 60 mgs daily

Masculini - T, herbal combination of muira puama, horny goat weed, maca, tribulus terrestris supports male hormone balance

Acetyl L-carnitine 1,000 mgs daily (stress/neuro-nutrient)

Vinpocetine - vasodilator, circulation

CoQ10 - heart health and circulation

Vitamin E - heart health

Maca Powder - adaptogen, hormone balance

Chrysin - passionflower for testosterone levels

Yohimbe (heart disease and diabetes), affects blood pressure and heart rate - 100 mgs

Panax Ginseng - endocrine system - 200 mgs

Testosterone Gel - prescription only

Chelation - DMPS (dimercapto propane sulfonate) and DMSA (dimercapto succinic acid)

Journaling - for stress and emotional processing

Homeopathic Staphysagria, Sepia

Mens primary health concerns are heart attack, cancer (especially prostate), diabetes and stress. Erectile dysfunction is often a symptom of advancing heart disease or cancer. Birth control and STD's are also men's health issues but are covered in the next chapter. Recovery from injury is the next most common health challenge for men. The process of recovery from injury is often a catalyst for recovery of overall general health.

SEXUALLY TRANSMITTED DISEASES

HPV - human papilloma virus is one of the most widespread of the venereal diseases and its longterm consequences can be devastating. Not only does it cause genital and anal warts, it can also cause warts in the throat and has been recently reassessed as the probable source of half of all oral cancers and the leading cause of cervical cancer and some anal cancers. The disease is dangerous and it is understandable to want a vaccine against it. There are two vaccines now available. The first was Gardasil, (available since 2006) which is formulated to protect against both warts and the viral related cancers that it causes. The newer vaccine, called Cevarix, claims to protect against cervical cancer and has not yet generated the negative public response that was expressed when many young woman appeared to be rapidly and permanently disabled shortly after receiving the original or first cervical cancer vaccine, or Gardasil.

Use of condoms for intercourse does not protect against transmission of the virus during oral sex. Homeopathy is the most effective therapeutic approach for clearing the virus from the body but homeopathy is notoriously slow and the process can be expected to take years.

Statistical analysis of the transmission of STD reveals that the risk factor for the individual rises dramatically in direct proportion to the number of sexual partners of both people. More partners means more diseases and some of them cause great suffering, disability and death. The ability to take realistic effective precautions against contracting and spreading sexually transmitted diseases and to take responsible action when STDs occur is a milestone of maturity that should precede becoming sexually active because failure to do so results in many cases of life long misery that are almost completely preventable.

HPV is just one of seven STD's that all sexually active people need to know how to protect themselves from as well as what to do if they may have been exposed. The most common STD's are herpes, hepatitis, chlamydia, gonorrhea, syphilis, HPV and AIDS (or HIV). Some of these diseases penetrate deep into the body, invading cells of the urethra, the fallopian tubes, the liver, kidneys, nerves and brain cells. These invasive diseases can be difficult to diagnose even when symptoms are apparent, but they often go undetected as their expression of symptoms is below the conscious level, and yet their silent damage produces infertility and cancer.

HPV

Viral, causes warts as well as thickening, cracking, and drying of skin. It particularly affects genitals, rectum and throat. It causes cervical dysplasia and cervical cancer. It is currently responsible for more cases of oral cancer than tobacco causes. The virus is considered to never be completely eradicated or cured, though warts can be removed. HPV is the number one risk factor in the development of cervical cancer which is the third most common cancer in women. Though the PAP test does not test for HPV, it does identify abnormal cellular changes called cervical dysplasia which is considered a precancerous condition caused by HPV infection.

Herpes

Viral, forms masses of small blisters which burst and form ulcerated sores which itch and burn and slowly scab over. The virus then becomes inactive but lies in wait in the nerve cells and re-emerges at times of physical depletion and stress. About 70% of adults have some form of herpes. About 45 million Americans have genital herpes.

Chlamydia

Bacterial, produces a deep infection of the fallopian tubes that is difficult to diagnose because current methods of testing have proved unreliable, frequently producing false results. The most common bacterial STD. About six million cases are diagnosed in the U.S. each year. The main organisms causing urethritis and cervicitis are chlamydia and gonorrhea. Symptoms are subtle but lead to serious complications including pelvic inflammatory disease (PID) and inflammation of the testes and prostate. Chlamydia causes infertility. It is treated with Doxycycline for two to four weeks. Also infects the throat, the rectum and the eyes.

Gonorrhea

Bacterial, is a leading cause of urethritis in both men and women. When untreated, it moves into deeper organs and produces infertility. It is penicillin sensitive and treated usually with a shot of penicillin but for those allergic to it, Ciprofloxacen may be given. Also infects the throat, the rectum and the eyes.

Syphilis

Bacterial, infects the blood and forms a lesion or ulcerated sore that will persist for a couple of weeks. Difficult to diagnose and often mistaken for other diseases. Treatment is antibiotics. It invades deeper tissue of bone, brain and spinal cord.

Hepatitis B and C

Viral, infects the blood, causes inflammation of the liver, nausea and general debility. It is easier to transmit than HIV, and can be passed in saliva. It causes scarring of the liver (cirrhosis) and liver cancer.

AIDS

Viral, infects the blood, also called HIV, causes immune deficiency and the patient ultimately dies of a series of subsequent infections against which the body has no defense. Maintaining overall general health with diet, exercise, supplements and stress management is the best treatment.

Candida

Candida is a yeast overgrowth infection which causes itching, red inflamed tissues that crack and split easily and a creamy discharge. It is due to sugar imbalance and common among diabetics and pre-diabetics. Candida infection of the vagina can be sexually transmitted but is often produced by overconsumption of sugars and highly refined foods or antibiotics. Treatment is vaginal anti-fungal cream or tablets and restricted diet. The candida diet severely restricts carbohydrates including sugars and starches, artificial sweeteners, yeast, alcohol, dry fruits and all processed foods

RECUPERATION, REBUILDING AND RECOVERY

Accidents, injury, surgeries and illness all require a period of recovery. Often that length of time is significantly greater than expected. Both the desire not to let one's life be disrupted and the assurance of one's doctor that recovery will be mundanely quick and easy lead to misunderstandings about what our healing process will require. These challenges often take about three times longer to resolve completely than what was anticipated.

When there is any underlying weakness hindering recovery, the amount of time needed to complete the healing increases. Underlying weakness includes high stress, which inhibits the immune response. Also factor in dehydration and acidosis. We look at these three weaknesses first because they are always made worse by any accident, trauma or illness. Both the challenge itself, as well as any medications and treatments, all increase the dehydration, acidosis and stress. Pre-existing underlying weakness that slows or prevents recovery includes both malnutrition and physical fitness.

Malnutrition is significant because there is so much rebuilding to do and the elements necessary for that reconstruction, from new blood cells to new tissue and bone healing are not readily available as needed. Physical fitness is revelant because circulation, oxygenation, metabolism and energy depend upon our capacity for sustained physical activity. If we are too weak or tired, then the body fails to produce enough CoQ10 to fuel the mitochondria, the basic energy of every cell.

Very often, there are underlying weaknesses that do not come to light until after an injury or illness has occurred. In other cases, such as a planned surgery, constitutional weakness may already be clearly apparent and be a predisposing factor for the surgery. Health that is maintained or symptoms that are controlled by medications, both prescription and non-prescription, indicates significant underlying weakness that can be expected to noticeably lengthen the time of recovery by weeks or even months.

Accidents that include broken bones or that require surgical repair increase the body's needs for nutrients, for hydration, for sleep and possibly other therapeutic modalities such as homeopathy, acupuncture and body work.

The degree to which these increased needs are met will determine the rate of healing. Trying to push through a recovery too soon or without attention to getting the body's real needs met is likely to produce an extended period of lingering lameness, weakness or debility. The liberal use of Floradix liquid vitamins is always well indicated to provide the support of super nutrition. Raw juice and broth are also recovery basics.

There is significant range of recovery times that varies from unexpectedly rapid to dismayingly slow. Rate of recovery also expresses something about honoring the meaningfulness of each challenge. Where our story about the event is upholding our positive self image, recovery will be much faster. To heal often requires that we discover how to creatively express our challenge in a positive light. Shifting the outlook to one that inspires, strengthens and upholds us, produces instantaneous healing. For example, I once received a call to provide support for a suspected attempted suicide.

While the patient was still comatose, I asked that his support team re-language this situation to eliminate implied criticism by referring to the event not as a suicide, but rather as a shamanic near death experience that was meant to happen for his benefit, instead of a terrible tragedy that should have been prevented. He was encouraged, upon returning to consciousness, to relax into the new set of circumstances without additional inner conflict of guilt or blame. Ultimately his experience provided a platform for his breakthrough to profound recovery of mental, emotional and physical health, happiness and creativity. The story used to define the experience (and the language) is part of the medicine, part of the recovery, or the story stands in the way of recovery and causes further wounding.

Healing from extreme traumas like murder, rape, shooting, stabbing, torture and violent crashes including cars, bikes and planes, generally takes about two years to reach a first level of recovery that includes diminished anxiety and reactivity to trauma triggers and increasing stability in day to day functions of self care, family life and eventually work. This plateau of recovery is metaphorically akin to the radioactive half life of this toxic exposure. Some degrees or types of traumas may persist for life though the individual is working through their own healing process. One doesn't heal such that it's as if you never had that experience. It will have it's influence, but one can shape and inform that influence with conscious intention of positive input and positive languaging to produce positive outcome and support healing.

Healing from grief is another form of trauma recovery. Processing deep grief can normally take anywhere from one to four years. In other cases, there is no recovery, and grief becomes a lifelong trial. Grief has both positive and negative forms of expression. There is a form of grief that makes fools of us all, that destabilizes us and robs us of all clarity, of even of the desire to live. Creating a positive form of expression for one's grief, establishing an endowment for charitable causes, addressing social problems and injustice with effective means for positive change or other personally meaningful creative expressions including songs, poems and stories or other art works takes the power of the wounding experience and uses it for transformation. Creatively engaging with one's grief resolves the negative emotional charge, whereas, avoidance and denial, which seemingly give one distance from grief, will cause that negative emotional charge to re-emerge at a later date when the possibility of processing to insight and healing is more likely.

Grief and trauma are also elements of acute and chronic illness. Pneumonia in particular and respiratory illness in general is directly triggered by grief. Full recovery from pneumonia and respiratory infections can take two to eight months depending upon both the degree of challenge to the overall health and upon the quality of the support system established. Other illnesses, including cancer, stroke and debilitating arthritis also generate grief and trauma because they may be both disabling and disfiguring.

Meningitis and encephalitis, infections of the spine or brain, can take four to nine months to recover even with optimal support in place. Recovery from mononucleosis also takes about five to nine months. Mono and pneumonia are both very prone to relapses, partial recovery, and lingering susceptibility to collapse.

Lyme's disease is another chronic acute illness that persists for months (usually 9 to 18 months) and which is characterized by lingering weakness and frequent relapses into episodes of acute symptoms, even when every effort to support recovery is well and insightfully attended to.

Recovering from joint replacement surgeries and organ removal (tonsils, gall bladder, uterus, prostate, spleen) is usually three to six months depending upon the overall general health and hydration going into the surgery as well as the quality of the support system for recovery. This is much longer, perhaps by several months, than may be suggested as the expected rate of recovery from these procedures by the medical practitioners that recommend and perform them. During the recovery process, the rate of healing is determined by the combination of the degree of injury or damage, the quality of the support system for recovery and the constitutional strengths and weaknesses, including physical, psychological and spiritual.

Essentially, everyone faces more than one of these extended episodes of recuperation in the course of a lifetime. Mastery of health and recovery of health play a role in the fulfillment of the purpose of life as it moves towards the perfection that it is divinely intended to manifest through the unfurling of the healing powers and potentials of the soul.

LED LIGHT THERAPY

The body is very responsive to light therapy and with high intensity LED lights we can get results that are as good as those achieved with much more expensive laser therapy. There are some surprises in light therapy and some aspects seem just as you would expect. Light therapy is beneficial for problems of brain atrophy such as in dementia, or pituitary problems, or in the limbic system and for PTSD. It is also beneficial for tissue regeneration and wound healing including surgeries and burns. It supports improved function in every organ and system of the body if hydration and pH are within normal range. It can be used to support heart health, respiratory health, and to overcome otherwise untreatable viruses like HPV and Herpes.

What surprises did I mean? I learned through working with the lights on my own body that blue light in through the chakras of the feet improves kidney health and in through the palms of the hands it improves thyroid function. Though I was not surprised that it was beneficial to put the therapy light into the chakras, I was surprised and delighted to note where that healing energy went. How long to use the light for each location varies with the individual and the location, but the most common is eight minutes, and the range is four minutes to twelve minutes per session. In most cases it would be used daily for the first three months and intermittently as needed after that. I provide specific instructions for each individual on what colors to use, on what locations, for how long and at what interval.

Blue LED

Blue LED light is the polychrest of light therapies. It has the most benefit for the greatest number of people and for the greatest number of the most common challenges. It is the light therapy color most beneficial for these problems: Brain atrophy, pituitary, pineal, limbic system, dementia, bi-polar depression and PTSD.

Ears, tinnitus, kidneys, adrenals, thyroid, teeth, bone marrow and blood (it increases erythropoietin levels to produce healthy red blood), aneurism, deep vein thrombosis, liver, spleen, gallbladder, osteoarthritis, chemical exposure to glyphosate, mercury, arsenic and silver (but not lead), mental health, addiction and anti-aging.

White LED

White LED light therapy is beneficial for prevention of heart attacks and treatment of them and also of respiratory weakness. Place in the center of the chest over the heart chakra. It is also supportive to healing the thymus, pancreas, ear infection and parasites.

Ultra violet LED

Ultra violet LED light therapy (purple) is beneficial for clearing viruses including HPV, HIV, shingles, herpes as well as flu and colds. It is also helpful for anemia, concussion (for coma use blue), rheumatoid arthritis, amputation, joint replacement, and chemical exposure to lead or carbon monoxide.

Green LED

Green LED light therapy is beneficial when combined with blue light therapy (at the same time not alternating blue and green) for drug and alcohol addiction, osteoarthritis and repetitive injury such as carpal tunnel. I love how the light therapy identifies addiction as a repetitive injury.

Red LED

Red LED light therapy is supportive to healing acne, rosacea, anti-aging of skin texture and fine wrinkles and for rosacea (combine with blue).

Only LED lights powered by lithium batteries will have the maximum therapeutic value. Non-lithium batteries are about 44% as effective for light therapy use.
Effectiveness of the light therapy also diminishes when the lithium batteries have discharged by 30%. Replace lithium batteries frequently to maintain therapeutic effectiveness.

HEALING TOUCH AND BODY WORK

Many readings recommend some form of healing touch or body work to support the recovery process. Massage is frequently recommended for those who cannot get enough physical exercise due to injury or illness. It is also recommended to improve circulation, lower blood pressure and promote relaxation because all of these benefits also produce improved immune functions. Massage is recommended for acute and chronic emotional stress because supportive touch also improves brain chemistry and mood. The three types of body work most frequently recommended are Cranio Sacral adjustments (an osteopathic modality), reflexology (pressure points on the feet) and deep tissue neuromuscular massage for release of negative emotional tensions and improved range of motion.

Reflexology is frequently recommended for kidney support, for lymphatic circulation and for blood circulation. It is particularly beneficial for those who are unable to be on their feet and physically active due to injury or illness however, it is also recommended for highly active but highly stressed individuals who may need support for balancing circulation, improving blood pressure and lowering cortisol levels. Painful areas on the feet correspond to areas of congested flow or blocked energy in other organs and systems of the body. Massaging and releasing these areas in the feet improves vital force through out the body. A series of a dozen reflexology sessions is usually recommended. It also relieves insomnia.

Clinical therapeutic massage is called deep tissue massage or neuro-muscular therapy. Trigger point massage and myotherapy are also included in this modality which is much more specialized than a gently relaxing Swedish massage. This deep tissue massage is at some point painful when trigger points are worked and may require conscious relaxation and co-operation to work through blockages. Doing so increases oxygen supply, lymphatic flow and the removal of waste and can be particularly helpful for bursitis, frozen shoulder, neck and back pain and headaches. When this form of body work is recommended in the medical intuitive readings, the usual suggestion is one session every 10 days for 3 to 6 session.

Cranio Sacral Therapy is frequently recommended in the readings as an effective support for the healing process that is gentle, subtle and holistic. The deep release and balance of flow in the body that is enhanced by this bio-mechanical adjustment improves overall well being by optimizing the functions of the central nervous system. When the flow of fluids and energies through the brain and spinal cord are optimal, support for and performance of every other organ in the body are improved.

This type of body work is not a massage. The client is fully dressed and lies comfortably on a padded table as the therapist moves around him/her and with a light touch assesses and adjusts areas of flow to relieve the source of weakness or dysfunction. Sessions are deeply relaxing. Recommended for headaches, neck and back pain, brain and spine injuries, nervous system weakness and PTSD.

ESSENTIAL OILS FOR SUSTAINABLE HEALTH
by Beret Jane Isaacson

Essential oils are a wonderful addition to a sustainable, healthy lifestyle. They are volatile liquids found in the flowers, bark, roots, seeds, and other parts of plants. They are obtained by steam distillation and have been used for thousands of years as medicine. Essential oils are being rediscovered by scientists as having numerous powerful healing benefits without the harmful side effects of synthetic drugs. Essential oils work at a cellular level and have a wide variety of applications in the realms of physical, mental, and emotional healing. They have antioxidant, antibacterial, antiviral, anti-infection, antimicrobial, antiseptic, antifungal, and anti-depressant properties. Essential oils may be used aromatically, topically, and internally.

A Note on Purity

Certified Pure Therapeutic Grade™ (CPTG™) essential oils from doTERRA provide the highest therapeutic value and are guaranteed free from harmful contaminants such as pesticides, herbicides, and any other chemical residues. The essential oil industry is not regulated, and it is legal to label as 100% natural and to sell essential oils that have been diluted with synthetic chemicals, alcohols, vegetable oils and other fillers. doTERRA CPTG™ essential oils are also tested to meet the standards of potency for the highest therapeutic effectiveness.

Aromatic

The aromatic use of essential oils is one of the most effective ways to treat mood and emotions. The limbic system of the brain includes the amygdala, which is a gland responsible for storing and releasing emotional trauma. The amygdala is accessed and stimulated via the sense of smell. When anxious or nervous, a calming oil like Roman Chamomile, Ylang Ylang or Lavender relaxes the nervous system. People suffering from depression will find support from any of the Citrus oils, Frankincense, Jasmine and Rose. To energize and focus, Peppermint and Rosemary are very invigorating to the body and intellect. People experiencing respiratory issues like colds, cough, pneumonia, bronchitis, and asthma can use the Respiratory Blend.

A diffuser is the best way to get the most aromatic benefit from essential oils. The AromaLite diffuser uses ultrasonic vibrations to disperse the essential oils and water together as a vapor. A few drops of essential oil will last for hours. It is also beneficial to put a drop of essential oil in the palm of your hand, rub your palms together, make a cup with your hands, and inhale. You can also inhale from the bottle. A few drops of Joyful Blend or Invigorating Blend as a natural perfume is another way to experience the aromatic benefits of the oils.

Topical

The largest pores of the body are on the soles of the feet. Essential oils applied to the bottom of the feet enter the bloodstream within 30 seconds and take about 20 minutes to travel throughout the entire body. Protective Blend boosts immunity, Peppermint cools the body or lowers a fever, and the Grounding Blend promotes a sense of balance and overall well-being.

Essential oils can have an immediate effect on the whole system when applied to the back of the neck at the base of the skull. Frankincense and Sandalwood contain natural chemical constituents called sesquiterpenes which are able to go past the blood-brain barrier, increase oxygen in the limbic system, positively affect the pineal and pituitary glands and lead to an increase in secretions of antibodies, endorphins, and neurotransmitters. Focus Blend, Calming Blend and Grounding Blend calm anxiety and tension, nourish the nervous system and support a positive outlook. Frankincense has anti-cancer, anti-depressant, and anti-inflammatory properties. Place 1 drop of Frankincense on the forehead, bottom of the feet or back of the neck every night at bedtime for healing support.

Many essential oils including Lavender can be used topically to treat a variety of skin conditions such as burns, cuts, rashes, bee stings, and ant and mosquito bites. Essential oils are also an important part of a repairing and anti-aging skin care routine. Some essential oils, like cinnamon, can be irritating to the skin and should be diluted with a carrier oil such as coconut oil, olive oil or jojoba oil. Products that are placed on our skin enter the bloodstream and affect not only our skin but our overall health and wellbeing.

Essential oils applied topically treat aches and pains, sore muscles and aching joints. doTERRA's Soothing Blend is analgesic and anti-inflammatory. It includes Wintergreen, Blue Tansy, German Chamomile, and Helichrysum. These penetrate deeply into muscles and joints. To provide soothing warmth, cover the area being treated with a snug woolen wrap, hot water bottle, or heating pad on low.

Essential oils can be used during prayer, meditation and yoga. Place a drop of Frankincense, Rose, Jasmine, Sandalwood, Myrrh or Joyful Blend over the heart, middle of the forehead, back of the neck, or bottom of the feet. Essential oils may also be diffused in the quiet space.

Internal

Be certain to use doTERRA CPTG™ essential oils. These are the only essential oils safe for internal use and are labeled as an Essential Oil Supplement with Supplement Facts when intended for internal use. These essential oils may be used in beverages and in cooking. In addition, a drop or two of an essential oil such as Peppermint or Digestive Blend can be used as oral hygiene or to treat digestive upset.

Place a drop or two of Lemon essential oil in your water every day. It will keep water bottles fresher longer due to their antibacterial effects. Make sure to use glass, ceramic, or 100% stainless steel, such as Kleen Kanteen, when adding essential oils to water because the oils will dissolve plastics. These same essential oils are able to do this in our bodies. All citrus oils break down petrochemicals in the body and cleanse and detoxify.

There are limitless ways to enjoy doTERRA essential oils in your foods and beverages. Enhance drink recipes with essential oils. To a quart of water add a drop of Lime essential oil and a handful of raspberries. In another quart of water add a drop of Peppermint and some sliced cucumbers, or a drop of Wild Orange and some strawberries. Add a drop of Cinnamon or Wild Orange to Fravarti's Bliss Ball recipes. Add 1 drop of Lemon or Lime essential oil to a fruit salad, a bowl of watermelon balls, or to a dressing for veggie salad. Try adding a drop of Peppermint or Wild Orange to chocolate recipes or to a bowl of ice cream. A little essential oil goes a long way. Often, 1 drop is enough for an entire recipe. If you desire less than 1 drop, you can insert a toothpick into the orifice reducer of your bottle to get just a little,and then stir it into your recipe. Experiment and enjoy certified pure therapeutic grade essential oils in your food and beverages.

Our senses can be deprived of natural sounds, colors, smells, tastes, and healthy touch. Likewise, our senses can be overstimulated by overactivity, tight schedules, screen time and long commutes. Essential oils can help with both deprivation and overstimulation. Try massaging your child's feet at bedtime with a drop of Lavender or Calming Blend. Diffuse an uplifting or calming blend into your living space. Experiment with the many nurturing ways to use essential oils and discover your favorites. The numerous powerful healing benefits of essential oils will enhance your life and the lives of those you love.

"Master aromatherapist Beret Jane is the creator of my favorite product MIRACLE SALVE and many other other fine personal care products. Contact her at beretjane.com".

Fravarti

ANTI - AGING

Anti-aging is written right into the divine plan. It is written in the epigenetic code of our DNA and it is part of the conscious intelligence of every cell of the body to preserve life, health and even youth. The intelligence of the body is working for the fulfillment of its purpose with every action that it takes. This intelligence of the body makes hundreds of thousands of choices, actions, or decisions at once, and it makes them all perfectly when operating within certain parameters of human physiology, including normal range of hydration, pH and nutrition. Other disrupters of this intelligence of the divine intention to heal are chemicals, especially those classified as biocides, and trauma which can be both physically and psychologically life threatening.

To support the body's innate conscious path of anti-aging and continuous restoration of its every organ, system, and function to ideal operational conditions and optimal health, the main objective would be to not work against this consciousness that is already pursuing and creating perfection on our behalf. First do no harm. Anti-aging means separating ourselves from the wide spread chemical exposure of processed convenience foods, the chemical exposure of packaging, preservatives, herbicides, insecticides, and personal care products including medications. It means living outside the convenience model that many have chosen and making different decisions to create different outcomes.

Getting off of medications is always a process of addressing the underlying reason for which the drug is used and changing the health such that the drug is no longer needed.

Some people will need to be on some medications for life and will not be able to discontinue certain prescriptions, even if they make all the best choices and accomplish all the healing that their body is capable of. However, letting your doctor know that you will do what it takes to be on as few medications as possible or even none eventually, helps them to understand how best to support you, which is quite different from what they must do to best serve and support those who will not make the changes that healing would require of them. The doctor can not presume the patient will begin making better choices than have been demonstrated thus far.

Planning long term for a long and healthy life is a good idea. Among those things most significant to that accomplishment would be to find your own pace. Most people are driven at a cultural pace, the pace of the expectations of the world and people around them. People are then driven by the pace of their own expectations, the ones they bought into when identifying with their culture, their peer's and their family's expectations. Balance in life and the lower stress level that comes with it are part of finding one's natural pace that allows for relaxing into ones life with whole hearted appreciation. Fear of the past and fear of the future promote a degree of efforting through out one's life that produces wear and tear by over extending beyond the capacities of the body. We call that wear and tear normal, but there is a mechanism of human design that minimizes and reduces wear and tear, and that is the balance of relaxation, rest and repose, together with physical and mental activity in the degree that is stimulating and productive of optimism and enthusiasm. This balance of finding one's natural pace that doesn't tear you down physically or psychologically creates happiness. Being observant and appreciative for what creates happiness is an excellent form of guidance for becoming truly oneself.

Those who have practiced yoga for thirty years often look about ten years younger than their peers who do not have a comparable practice of some sort. That's because long term practice of yoga contributes not only to physical fitness, stamina and resilience, it also supports balance, mental clarity, happiness and lower stress levels. The practice of yoga is proven to help with back pain and weakness, with heart health and with developing core strength. Its an anti-aging power house and the cute little outfits are strictly optional. You don't even need to leave home to practice. All you need is a body, breath and consciousness.

Beyond the balance of activity and repose, to optimize stress levels, one of the most important considerations reflective of and supportive of overall general health is oral dental health. Ten years of aging can easily be added by neglect of oral health and ten years of anti-aging can be gained by excellence in dental hygiene together with needed repairs and reconstruction. Removing all the teeth and replacing them with dentures is more aging to the body than putting in implants and replacing and repairing teeth as needed. Getting the very best dental work is more valuable than getting the very best price.

As to its anti-aging benefits, a good dental reconstruction (that may include implants and veneers) can be more valuable than a ten thousand dollar face lift. Not only do our teeth age us visually by their appearance but they also age us physically and psychologically. They have a profound impact on our self image and confidence. They do so because they have a similarly profound effect on how others see us and respond to us. Make oral health a key note of your anti-aging lifestyle.

The happiness of living a life you want to live, a life that rewards you for being you, creates an abundance of youthful vitality. Living a life that generates an experience of feeling like you would rather die is not a life affirming, health promoting path. The ability to make changes in ourselves and in our lives to create greater happiness both for ourselves and for those around us is the essence of spiritual wisdom and insight, and it is the much sought fountain of eternal youth. We die when we don't want to live. We die when living suppresses or denies us.

Letting go of the life that is killing you, of the life that robs you of your energy and enthusiasm and depletes your joy, is the way to die daily to the limitations of physical embodiment and to awaken more fully into the consciousness of immortality. In pursuit of connection with the consciousness of immortality, I recommend deepening and developing ones conscious relationship with the Sun, in which we live and move and have our being. The early morning light is prized for its benefits through the practice of Sun-gazing. This ancient practice is very powerful for stimulating the pineal gland and awakening its perception of connectedness to the universe and an innate guidance as a being of light on a path of endless light. The practice is best begun at the moment of dawn when the sun begins to rise above the horizon. The sun's rays are the most gentle and least damaging for those first three to five minutes of the day. Place the fingers of both hands in front of the face, cross wise to each other to form a lattice work.

Look between the fingers while adjusting them to form a pin hole that blocks out the corona of the sun, the outer edge, and directs the gaze to the central sun. Allowing this light to fall upon and be absorbed by each eye for two minutes four times a week maximizes the anti-aging benefits of this practice and supports illumination of the mind as well as improved brain functions.

In further developing a personal relationship with the sun, seek out its light during those hours of the day that it is most beneficial. Yes, avoid sunburn. Yes, avoid over exposure at the wrong time of the day. But sunlight is as beneficial as air and water. It is essential to the health of every cell of the body and supports healthy skin, healthy gut where vitamin D is produced and healthy bones where vitamin D promotes healthy mineralization and bone strength. Twenty minutes of early morning light five days a week reads very high as an anti-aging practice. This concentration of receiving the benefits of morning light can be combined with a passion for gardening or invigorating exercise. Don't miss out on the benefits of morning. It has anti-aging powers galore.

Recovery from accidents, injury, trauma, surgery and illness all play a prominent role in the experience of aging. For one patient, all weakness or complaint is seemingly subsequent to some specific challenge; whereas, for another, the real recovery and reclaiming of able bodied wellness comes about as a response to one of those challenges, finally providing the motivation to do what works. Recovery from any one of these challenges takes longer and is less than optimally realized when steps are not taken to meet all the real needs involved. Accident, injuries, surgeries and illness all disrupt hydration and pH due to shock, trauma, cortisol and adrenalin. Medications and anesthesias also reduce pH and hydration. Not addressing the challenge to hydration will slow or prevent full recovery. Additionally, healing is nutritionally demanding. The raw materials must be available in a form that is well matched to the challenge and may require supplements and a therapeutic diet. Lack of the essential building blocks will delay or prevent full recovery.

Taking the time for full recovery from injury, surgery and illness also means taking time for both exercise and rest. These two pillars are essential to rebuilding health. Exercise to build strength and vitality, to support circulation and efficient detoxing, to improve metabolism and cognitive functions, must also be balanced with increased rest and sleep. The body heals twice as fast when asleep. Recovery requires extra sleep, usually together with extra exercise. Failure to invest enough of either one of these to the full degree that the challenges require will also delay or even prevent full recovery.

The challenge of accidents, surgeries and illness will happen in every life. In many cases, that challenge will initiate changes that become a foundation for anti-aging. Take the time and interest to address the full spectrum of need for recovery to restore and maintain youthful wellness and vitality. Don't stay broken. Instead, use the break-down, whether injury or illness, to validate your real needs and make healing choices. It will keep you young.

Nine Steps To Anti-Aging

Balance - Lower stress level, finding a natural pace allows hormone and psychological balance. Relaxing into life instead of promoting wear and tear. Use body work, massage, exercise, yoga, rest, relaxation, self examination and meditation.

Happiness - Self concept is the basis of happiness. Who you are, not what is happening to you, is the source of happiness. Be the person you want to live with forever. Meditation, immortality, meaningfulness, prayer, journaling, calling or service work.

Exercise - Fitness, stamina, resilience, flexibility. Promotes circulatory health, heart health, brain health, sleep and positive self image.

Rest - Refreshed, energized, restored. Sleep, naps, meditation, day dreaming, contemplation, pause.

Diet - Nutritional excellence, alkaline pH, super hydration, low toxic burden.

Chemical Exposure - Chemicals cause cell death and mutation, reduced chemical exposure environmentally, as well as through diet and medication promote the natural anti-aging abilities of the body.

Sun Gazing and Proper Sunbathing - Support for the pineal gland and production of vitamin D. promotes light in the outlook and healthy skin.

Accidents, Injuries, Surgeries and Illness - Recovery from these challenges and implementing the changes required by them, including taking enough responsibility for self care, and getting all your needs met.

Oral and Dental Health - Excellent hygiene and repairs promote anti-aging.

ECONOMY AND HEALTH

57% of people recently surveyed say that the economy has affected their health care choices (Parade Magazine 5/17/09). People report that they are choosing to skip flu shots, mammograms, routine physicals, anti-cholesterol drugs, dental cleanings and psychotherapy sessions. Our current health care system is broken because it pays for emergencies (exorbitantly) and places no emphasis on responsibility for prevention of disease and the deliberate conscious creation of health. Preventative efforts reduce hospitalizations and prescription costs and cost much less than crisis intervention. Some people have reported that they are choosing to skip fresh fruits and vegetables (30%) and using the economy as their excuse - i.e., too expensive. They would be better served by skipping the non-nutritive foods (chips, pasta, pastry, crackers, candy, cookies, soda, alcohol) and spend more on whole fresh foods to create optimum health and immunity.

WISE WAYS TO LOWER COSTS / UNWISE WAYS TO SAVE MONEY

Exercise - 30 to 60 minutes daily build stamina and resilience	DON'T skip exercise - and do fix your bike, buy a trampoline, join a fitness center
Whole fresh Organic food keep that 6.6 pH balance	DON'T buy cheap food, (eat real not fake food)
Use supplements wisely	DON'T skip needed supplements
Drink water, lots of water	DON'T skip Penta if your hydration is below 3
Detox the body & avoid pesticide & toxic exposures	DON'T skip alternative health support, visit your N.D., D.O., acupuncturist, chiropractor, body work therapists of all kinds
Get off prescriptions when you can. Ask your doctor to help you reduce your prescriptions	But DON'T quit w/o making necessary changes to overcome cholesterol, hypertension, etc. and check with your doctor.

Rest, meditate, pray, lower stress, take retreats, & rebalance frequently

DON'T skip getting together w/ loved ones and be generous always

Practice gratitude and forgiveness

DON'T skip your Spiritual Tithe. Never tell yourself you can't afford to give anything. There are always those who have even less.

Control your weight

DON'T tell yourself it doesn't matter. It does.

Quit smoking

Quit or reduce alcohol

Brush, floss & clean your own teeth

THE ECONOMICS OF NATURAL HEALING

What does it cost to work with me as a medical intuitive? Most patients initially spend between $500.00 and $1,000.00 per year for my consultations. They may spend an additional $600.00 to $700.00 annually on supplements and remedies. Additional therapeutic modalities are often recommended including body work, counseling, IV therapies, hyperbaric treatments and exercise classes and equipment. The upgraded diet costs an average of $700.00 in additional expense each year. To do everything I recommend can cost $3,000.00 per person some years, but when intravenous chelation is required or a drug detox treatment with Ibogaine is needed, the price can easily soar to ten thousand dollars. The healthier one is when we start, the less it costs to meet their health goals.

My practice would be rather elitist if I served only those who can pay these prices. The truth is that with some clients I have bartered, an exchange of my work for theirs. For some clients, I have waved my fees altogether and occasionally, when it has been my spiritual calling to do so, I even provided the remedies, the supplements and some of the food from my own pocket book. I feel privileged to feed people and consider it a primary spiritual practice. My work as a medical intuitive is also my spiritual practice. It is based in meditation and prayer just as much as it is grounded in training and experience. Most clients learn from my expertise and are able to reduce their dependency on guidance very quickly. Revealing why each recommendation is made fosters future independence and self-reliance based on clear insight and understanding. It also provides very strong reality based motivation to do what works to create the desired outcome.

I have said that some clients spend several thousands dollars, maybe for a few years, to achieve their health and wellness goals. Compared to not spending anything, that can seem like a lot of money. Compared to the $100,000.00 treatments offered by modern medicine, compared to heart attacks and diabetes, cancer, dementia and joint or organ replacement, the cost of working with me and doing all that natural healing requires is really the least expensive path in every way.

Over the course of 25 years and over 30,000 consultations, Fravarti has answered almost a million questions for doctors and clients. In clear concise language she provides practical insights as to what does and does not work in restoring vibrant health. Now everyone can more readily achieve their health and healing goals while avoiding spending money on popular products and marketing miracles that cannot fulfill their claimed potentials and won't produce the needed results.

HAPPINESS AND THE PSYCHOLOGY OF HEALTH

Happiness is the natural state of the soul and to enjoy a state of happiness confers a degree of God realization, an aligning of the personal outlook in harmony with the divine. A happy person is in harmony with the life he lives even when facing challenges of pain and difficulty. True happiness is common in children under the age of seven. After that, happiness can seem fleeting or elusive due to cultural conditioning of learned dissatisfaction and the development of the critical outlook which builds defenses for the ego out of seeing what's wrong in any situation and whose fault it is.

Happiness is a no fault policy, an outlook of non-judgmental observation that does not sort everything into good or bad and right or wrong. Our attachment to our conditioned beliefs, which includes the limitations we incorporate into the self concept as to what weaknesses, failing and shortcomings we identify with, is a great source of unhappiness to us. Much more so than our actual conditions in life, our belief about those conditions and about what those conditions should be will determine how much happiness we are experiencing. We tell ourselves things are bad, people are bad, and circumstances are unbearable, and we experience all to be exactly as we have described it.

We can develop, in time and with deliberate practice, the ability to step back from our judgments, to renounce our criticisms as not particularly valid or valuable and thereby more easily cultivate a greater general happiness in our lives by not habitually setting ourselves in conflict with what is - or appears to be. Happiness is, for adults who face ongoing stress, a choice of intentional resilience, adaptability and grace under pressure. Unhappiness, in the form of fear, depression or pessimism produces a brittle, crisis oriented, alarmist outlook and an inflexibility due to one's judgments and expectations that produces disaster again and again. Being unhappy, critical, fearful, or pessimistic is a learned choice that originates from lack of trust in one's self and in one's environment and one's experience or of people and even of the Creator. One who can not trust himself cannot trust anyone and cannot trust that there is reason to be happy or that it is safe or wise to do so. While experiencing unhappiness, one tends to support it with the inner stance that it would be crazy not to be unhappy.

So far so good. At this point begins the experience we call a dark night, a process that invites re-orienting, which could also be called soul retrieval, a re-orienting such that the new outlook entices your soul back into the dance of your life. Depression when looked at this way is not so much about the chemical imbalance that has developed, but rather it is a beneficial response from the intelligence of the body. Observing a fruitless situation, it shuts down to conserve energy and wisely refuses to invest it's resources. It's message is: "Change or die."

What we believe determines what we feel and invests our experience with meaningfulness. Change what we believe, change what we are doing that creates unhappiness and do more of what creates happiness and we change not only our experience outwardly but also our self concept. Who we have conceived ourselves to be becomes more empowered, resilient and sturdy against what life can require of us. The soul is immortal, invincible and irrepressible. Any contact with the soul exalts one's being. How does one call forth the soul? With passion and deep commitment to use the time and opportunities given to you to relentlessly pursue your own happiness as well as your ability to create happiness in the lives of those around you.

Mastering your ability to change what you think and what you feel is an essential life skill. The wisdom of how to do exactly that has been passed down for thousands of years and has been a part of spiritual training and practice for all peoples in all times. The fast track to changing how you feel starts with the intention to do so. Next put awareness on the breath and put the intention to change and change to what on the breath. Slow the breath and stay present to the intention you choose. Sometimes you can re-center, balance and find your point of power all on one breath. Sometimes it takes ninety-nine breaths. Do what it takes. For those experiencing intractable anxiety, conscious breath practices together with proper hydration are the most effective therapy. They may work better than prescription medications.

Change your environment so that it accommodates and supports you, providing comfort, rest, sustenance and a sense of well-being. The conditions of the environment carry clues and messages as to our own condition. Going out in nature changes the message and is one of the fastest, surest ways to do so. The sky, the sun and the stars evoke a larger outlook and reaffirm a grander scope of purpose and glory. A walk in the woods helps us reconnect with the stateliness of our own being and nurtures our sense of liberty, inspiration and satisfaction.

The biblical injunction to first set thine own house in order is a significantly helpful guideline about taking personal responsibility for the space and energy within which you live, move and have your being. This means inside your home as well as inside your body and even in the subtle bodies. Setting thine own house in order includes emotional sorting and getting over it. Choose resilience, peace and happiness because you can and because it is wise to do so. Sorting and cleaning the environment, laundry, dishes and clutter is conducive to sorting one's thoughts and emotions.

Water in any form, is beneficial to promoting happiness. Drinking water or a cup of tea lowers anxiety. Relaxing beside water in streams, fountains, lakes, rivers and oceans and even more so, relaxing in the water, including baths, showers, hot tubs and pools, is very soothing and nurturing and can change one's entire outlook in just a few minutes.

Choosing appropriate music to create feelings of happiness or uplifting emotions is a very powerful support for a healthy outlook and often provides needed relief from persistent unwanted thoughts or worries. Well chosen music stimulates an increase in the release of dopamine and endorphins. Singing, dancing, yoga and other forms of connecting with the creative, expressive self have a reassuring effect on the psyche and become very empowering when regularly practiced every day over the long term.

It is also helpful to create a "do" list of tried and proven ways to create positive emotions. Make a things I like to do list when you are happy and well balanced enough to notice all the many things that support and contribute to your happiness. Then in those dark night moments when you are telling yourself you don't remember how to be happy and have forgotten what you love, go back to the list and choose some of the many things that have worked for you before.

Jesus summarized this point about attitude and outlook quite succinctly: "My yoke is easy, my burden is light." His statement highlights the spiritual power and specifically the light of a positive attitude. Further elucidation of this point can be found in His statement "give them your cloak also", suggesting an orientation or outlook that instead of worrying that one has been robbed, will turn it around in the mind and make it more beautiful by the power you have to put a positive spin on things, relenting of judgment and criticism and indulging in appreciation, gratitude and wonder. Don't choose to have a bad time by telling yourself things are not good. Continually re-injuring oneself by rehashing the past as a negative, undesirable experience is a way of keeping one's woundedness (ego) alive and honoring one's woundedness above one's ability and responsibility to heal.

The story, the history, which you believe about your woundedness and the injustice in your life, is not really true. The mind has added up the available facts and come to the wrong conclusion. It is full of distortion and misinformation and holds you back by requiring much of your energy and identity to be tied up in maintaining and honoring your version of your story. When you are able to observe your negativity, deny it some degree of validity. Step back from it, soften it, and begin to construct a mental version that's not about honoring the story that you have carried up to this point, but is about creating a better story that can heal you and carry you towards spiritual liberty, illumination and realization. When we lose sight of our happiness, we have to choose happiness again.

It seems likely that the greatest impediment to human happiness has long been the tendency towards the critical outlook: judging ourselves as not good enough, judging others as not what they should be and circumstances as intolerable. Eating of the fruit of the tree of knowledge of good and evil is still getting us kicked out of paradise today. We don't generally criticize our newborns, but at some point, early on, we begin to tell children that there is something wrong with them and they will have to change, improve, and come up to expectations or be judged not good enough and suffer the consequences of being thrown out of the garden. By age seven, most children are well trained to walk into any situation and determine what's wrong and whose fault it is. We teach them to look for what is wrong in life and tell them that doing so will keep them out of trouble by providing knowledge and maybe evidence (at least circumstantial) to prove that someone else is at fault, the fall guy, the one to blame.

But really there are no bad guys except for those occasions where the good guys are also the bad guys. We are all in this together and everyone is good and everyone is imperfect and will have their moments of manifesting that weakness or flaw. When your experience seems to victimize you, look for the subtle ways in which you participate in manifesting this dynamic. One may have the same experience thousands of times and yet not choose the victim role every time. Sometimes we refuse to take it on. We refuse to go there and we mentally distance ourselves from the situation that could be seen as victimizing, not allowing someone's rudeness, carelessness or even injustice to really get to us. We don't take it on every time and when we do, we have chosen our victimizer or person to blame very carefully. We choose, at some level of our beings, which moments and which people to react to. And at other times we choose indifference in response to the same affront or challenge.

We can learn to choose indifference, spiritual detachment, almost every time once we decide and set the intention that we will control our experience by controlling our reactions, rather than by controlling others or circumstances. The lament: "I would be okay, if only he, she or it would change." is a trap, a position of powerlessness. That outlook makes whether or not you will be victimized appear to lie in someone else's control and not in yours. It keeps one from taking responsibility for changing what you can and creates resentment through acting out control dramas to try to manipulate or influence others to get the preferred outcome.

Happiness requires learning to make peace with what is, softening the outlook. In many cases, this means you yourself contributing all the beauty that seems otherwise lacking just by refusing to criticize or condemn. One does not become a spiritually illuminated, God realized human being until one is able to overcome grudges against people, overcome the tendency to blame and to resentment, hatred, jealousy and intolerance. Powerful luminous emotions of compassion and generosity will make you radiant.

A common weakness undermining our happiness is the almost universal desire to have an advantage and to call that state of apparent advantage being okay. This means that being neutral, balanced and fair is not okay and is less desirable, certainly less secure. This is a fear based illusion which promotes an outlook of entitlement and greed. There is nothing for sale in the marketplace of the world for less than full price. Do not be deceived. Do not willingly deceive yourself. Putting someone at a disadvantage never makes you more okay. Making things easier on yourself by making things harder on someone else always leaves the impression of a wounding presence on one's sense of justice.

It is hard to identify with the nobility of the soul if your motives and actions don't look very noble, even to yourself. To let another suffer more so that you might suffer less is not a courageous response to life's challenge. If you are conditioned to believe that your well-being and perhaps even your very survival are dependent upon circumstances being not just, fair or balanced, but rather upon getting something for less than it's worth or for free because you fear not being okay enough or gratified enough when paying full value and full price, then you have bought into the cultural con that is using you and using us all in an imbalanced and narcissistic way that is not sustainable.

Talk yourself out of this nonsense. The welfare of others is always a consideration. It makes you and your loved ones unhappy to always be trying to get more for less ~ less time, less money, less resources and less care. The premise that it's okay for you to have less so that someone else can have more is a constant fear nagging at our self image and our confidence. No matter which side of the equation one is on it robs you of any sense of nobility.

The greatest power for achieving happiness and the greatest strength for maintaining it comes from believing that you don't need any additional advantages because the divine inheritance in your own being is the only advantage anyone has ever needed, and you can never be separated from that holy power which is creating all things.

We can experience the happiness in our own being more deeply, consciously and profoundly when we choose to rebalance and center throughout each day, intentionally returning to the place where happiness abides - in hope, faith, trust, confidence, love, honor, and the many divine qualities that constitute our essential self, our grandest most glorious version of self that we can conceive. Happiness through advantages in business, pleasure and entertainment, or in relationships is not a stable, reliable form of happiness. Happiness in who you know yourself to be, even if no one else cares, is a mastery that cannot be taken from you.

If you are not happy, truly happy, despite life's challenges, start making changes in who you choose to be and what you choose to do, think, eat, drink, and how you schedule your time, which of your weaknesses you choose to indulge or not, which of your abilities or strengths you develop more completely and express your passion through. Then change these things as necessary again and again until you come to all those little solutions that work for you, that support, uphold and encourage you. To have life more abundantly, look at what fills you with optimism, enthusiasm, energy and courage to take your next step and consider that a form of spiritual guidance to have and do those things in your life. Notice also when something depletes you of joy, energy and enthusiasm. It's not enough to just say: "I don't want to live this experience. It's killing me." If it's killing you, the It is you. Stop and do what you love and more of what you think you might love and when you don't love it anymore, choose again. Stay authentic.

The Universe does not require that you do those things that rob you of your joy and deplete your will to live. The Universe is giving you the privilege of the freedom to choose to do or be anything you want, anything at all. If you can imagine it and intentionally choose to commit to creating your next grandest version of you and of your possibilities, of your life and what you would like to be, then life's continuous struggles become imbued with a deeper meaningfulness as your small share of the birth pangs of the Universe unfurling its infinite glory. The glory of your soul is an extension or a part of that glory that is the Universe. Your soul is immortal, powerful, and irrepressible. Living the life of your soul will create sustainable happiness in life and that happiness will make you healthier and wiser.

You do not have to live a life of misery if you learn to practice taking control of how you feel, what you think, and of your reactions and you can learn to tell a better version of your story ~ One that heals you, supports you, and upholds you. Put a positive spin on things because it is a great power to be able to do so. Quit the job of being unhappy, a martyr, afraid, inadequate and insecure. Pick a new job. Develop your talents and abilities. Be invincible and irrepressible by identifying with that in you which is greater than your small self. Die to what is not serving you and resurrect now, creating new possibilities of realization and mastery. Become the embodiment of happiness and do it deliberately by overlooking all that would distract you from that happiness and by remembering to be intentionally present to the authentic source of happiness in one's own being. No one can make you happy. You do it to yourself. Dare to do what it takes for you to be happy, including change your beliefs, your values, and your self concept as well as what you do with your time. Do it because by that process you make yourself strong, resilient, beautiful, and a blessing both to yourself and in the lives of those around you.

"Happiness is the consequence of personal effort...You have to participate relentlessly in the manifestations of your own blessings".

Elizabeth Gilbert

MASTERY IN THE DARK NIGHTS

Sometimes knowing the right answer about what best supports our health and well being is not enough. The psychological challenge of grief, loss and despair usually undermine our ability to make the wisely guided choice. In the dark night of the mind or the dark night of the soul, when the mantra of "I don't care" rises unbidden in every moment, we become unable to care for ourselves, even when we know what it would take and exactly how to do it.

The whole, natural food in our refrigerator mocks us as it slowly decays. They seem to represent our own natural health and wellness deteriorating as we reach past the organic cage free eggs and the watermelon to grab the least healthy treat we can find - chocolates or puddings, wheat, sugar and unhealthy fats. These empty calories that will make us as physically distressed as we feel psychologically, are the only things we are eating - deliberately starving ourselves of any real nutritive support. We eagerly consume everything that represents rebellion. We continue feeding ourselves lies, mentally and physically until our inner sickness manifests the imbalance outwardly, forcing us to change or die, perhaps slowly with great suffering to express our inner vision and self concepts.

We are habitually eating as if we are dying and each moment is another opportunity to savor that special treat as if it were our last meal ever (and yes, it will kill you - but slowly and you're dying everyday anyway so you think "at least I can have this"). I'll still be dying but enjoy it more, or at least seem to for a moment of sweet relief from the burden of despair.

Eventually, something opens our wings and inspires us to live instead of die. Some flicker from the depth of our immortal being reminds us that we don't die, really. Even that which kills us does not really kill us. Yes, I know you can not bear it because you are a limited human being pushed beyond your capacity - but do it anyway because life goes on forever. It never ends. You learn never to need anything so badly that you can't live without it - because that isn't real. You live forever, with or without whatever. You rise to the challenge as if there is nothing that can't be done and you begin to meet life on its own terms.

The solution to your challenge is always in you being more authentic, be yourself, be real. Then you can begin to get more of your real needs met and create a stronger support system for the happiness that is the true nature of the soul; irrepressible, resilient and courageous. Yes, we get off track, overindulge and rebel, but we also start again and change things as we can and take personal responsibility again and again until we master the insights of what works to sustain and uphold, us, to heal and inspire us and what depletes us of those strengths.

Life is what it is, and the dark nights will come around again. We will get off track again and need to make our way back. We can learn to pay attention to our own cycles and observe honestly where we are out of balance and start with intention. Intention to do what we can to enjoy the privilege of life itself with all its darkness of every kind, still, it is also full of wonder just by shifting one's attention to deliberately wonder about the glory of the cosmos, the stars and galaxies, the mysteries of creation and the power of love. The mind can participate in our upliftment and create landscapes of light and beauty that entice our souls to participate in the dance of life with us, filling us with invincible irrepressible spirit - which is the nature of both the soul and of life itself.

The mind can support us in creatively and brilliantly changing our story to one that better supports us and upholds us. The mind can provide deeper meaningfulness to grief and loss as our pain is reinterpreted and becomes our share of the birth pangs of the self we are choosing to be now, a new self, vibrant with life affirming energies that emerge from the darkness that has been transformed by the power of the human heart into all things light. Change your story, your self concept, and your experience of life also changes. Our stories aren't really true so please change yours to one that better supports you and upholds a positive self image and aligns you with a positive concept of life in the present moment.

These cycles are normal. We are not always at the top of our game. When we find ourselves in a dark night process it is best to have a plan based on everything that has worked before, as to how we might best manage all that this experience can require of us. Conscious relaxation techniques, centering prayer and yoga can all support moving into balance and clarity. If you are challenged and distressed enough to be disabled and dysfunctional, it would be best or ideal to stop functioning (or pretending to) in the mundane spheres of life and retreat for some inner process work, self examination and journaling.

Even a half day mini retreat, maybe a nap, a bath, soulful solitude or joyful music, a walk in nature, can be enough to shift one's energy and outlook from can't to can and from frazzled to fine. However, the challenge of the dark night can persist even for years, and when that is the case, a longer retreat process may be called for to support the transformation that is needed. A qualified retreat guide can help design an experience that heals and upholds you in unfurling your life's purpose and the realization of your personal goals for health and wellness as well as clarity and confidence. Dark night experiences are meant for our benefit. They are the ultimate motivation for change and transformation of one's experience and one's interpretation of life's challenges and privileges. They influence us to stop doing what isn't working.

"... and men are, that they might have Joy."

2 Nephi 2:25

"There is no medicine as powerful as Joy."

Leo Buscaglia

SELF - ESTEEM

To study and understand self-esteem we will look at five different aspects or frequencies. All self-esteem frequencies overcome aspects of fear. Self-esteem is essential to the fulfillment of the purpose of life, realization. When deeper examination of the self concept is necessary, one can practice a careful study of different aspects of the personal identity or self image which are the foundation of healthy self-esteem including cultivating awareness of our inner nobility, our deepest and best self, and the holder of our ideals of chivalry.

The self-esteem of knowing the nobility of the soul confers modesty and overcomes shame. It also supports intuition and leads one towards making noble choices in life. The quality of nobility, specifically the Nobility of the Divine Being, is the fabric of the soul; is the light of glory shining out of each being which shows the purpose of his life. This light in man proves his purpose which is the creation of beauty, the beauty of illumination, the illumination of the truth - which is the answer to every question and the solution to every problem. What the soul needs is knowledge of itself, so that it is not deluded by experiencing the life of the body and of the mind. One's real being is not dependent upon external validation for its identity, but is the light of life itself, immortal, all-pervading, and silent, yet communicates with all life in the universal language of vibrations. The nobility of the soul is a treasure that endures forever, a light that will never be extinguished and that guides one to the fulfillment of life's purpose.

Self-esteem includes feeling above reproach, innocent and pure with a sense of natural appreciation. The self-esteem of not feeling criticized confers balance in self-esteem and overcomes low self-esteem and fear of rejection, and not being good enough by knowing what is truly praiseworthy about oneself while not being afraid to make (and own) mistakes.

A noncritical outlook towards self and others (you can't get it wrong) overcomes vulnerability to praise and blame. Self-esteem is grounded in the personality while striving to better oneself by refraining from ever doing those things of which you personally disapprove. Remembering that your own self witnesses all that you do, knows when you are honorable and invariably condemns you when you are not, actually supports both strong stable self-esteem and honorable behaviors.

The emotion of being above reproach is the feeling we get when we witness a rainbow and the natural evocation of OH's and AH's that rise from the heart in response. Every rainbow one sees is beautiful and appreciated even if it is incomplete or indistinct. Even rainbows that are but weak intimations of the full rainbow potential are still valued and not criticized.

The self-esteem of feeling special or unique in a valuable way confers Self-Realization and overcomes hate and rebelliousness. It is an ability to self-validate that comes from an unshakable knowing that you are very good at what you do. It is for this purpose that we are born. What is special or unique about oneself gives one a way of living in self-esteem that is non-judgmental and defuses the inevitable situations of human error and relaxes the defense system to a receptive mode that can accommodate the imperfections without threatening the uniqueness or specialness which support our self-esteem. The self concept of being valuable anyway, in fact a treasure, despite our limitations, is essential to strong stable self-esteem. Divine creativity is customized as individual creativity as one imagines what they wish to become and actively incorporates that into the unfurling of the personality.

The self-esteem of feeling equal to whatever life can require of you confers courage and overcomes the sense of personal inadequacy (and the identity of 'underachiever'). It is a strong psychological defense and overcomes the sense of things not being fair, not equitable. Being able to respond from a place of balance to a situation that is out of balance and thus restore balance within and without. Every reason that you have for why you are not yet all that you could be - there is nothing unfair about it. This is simply the process that allows you to unfurl the potentialities of your being by challenging you to evolve and perfect yourself in response to circumstantial limitation and knowledge born of experience. You actuate the splendor of your soul when you rise to this challenge. Your dependence on circumstances being as you like is just like an addiction. We do not need freedom from circumstances. What we need is freedom from our conditioning. Our creativity is our freedom. We can recreate ourselves in a way that makes our experience work for us.

The self-esteem of realizing you can have whatever you want and do what ever you want, no dream too great to go after (To Dream the Impossible Dream) confers God-Realization and overcomes weakness of pride and revulsion. This realization leads to an intuitively guided life of divine inspiration. Self-esteem promotes a quality of adaptability or the functional concept of oneself as highly adaptable due to one's strengths, particularly the strength of being greater than one's obstacles as an integral part of one's self concept. The resources of one's being that one has to bring to bear upon one's problems is almost unlimited - immeasurably great. Whatever one wants, it is within his potentials and possibilities to have it, with no exceptions. It begins with the ability to see the stepping stones to success in failure and it produces the awareness of having at one's disposal all that is necessary to solve one's problems.

The concept that nothing is too good to be true or too wonderful to happen promotes the courage to be who ever you want to be, the courage to be authentic, which is self- esteem.

"If you wish to be a warrior prepare to get broken, if you wish to be an explorer prepare to get lost and if you wish to be a lover prepare to be both."

Daniel Saint

BOUNDARY STYLES

In doing attunements to oneself and others (readings), it can be very helpful to distinguish three basic boundary styles which are the defenses of the false ego. Every person uses all three styles, at different times, to access their God given right to avoidance and denial as defenses of the ego. Each of us has a dominant style but will resort to one of the other two if it seems more likely to produce the result we want than the one we have been using. Each style has specific health manifestations that may be linked to it. All three styles produce frequencies that result in dehydration, liver disease and dementia.

Narcissism

"It's all about me". You are an extension of me; one of my resources or assets.

Hidden contract or agenda: You will benefit by benefitting me (supposedly) but it is not up to me to look out for you specifically. Your benefit is presumed to be an automatic side effect of my benefit.

Personality development: aspects of failed individuation with infantile features family history of alcoholism, addiction, and chronic illness including but not limited to mental illness, cancer, MS, CF, CP, epilepsy, diabetes - or anything else that constantly overrides any other consideration by presenting in acute and alarming crisis again and again - predisposes to the narcissistic personality because the infant or child does not get real needs met and does not move completely out of the infantile state of cognizance of how to get those needs met.

The narcissist needs to learn COMPASSION, learn to care about the experience of the person you are exploiting. When you let consequences that should fall on you shift onto someone else, you fail to take responsibility in the way that will lead to mastery.

Narcissism manifests as dehydration outside the cell wall in the interstitial fluid which impairs elimination and lymphatic function and produces rising toxic levels. They develop heart disease, diabetes, COPD, and other diseases that make them the center of the universe (including addictions).

Co-Dependence

"It's all about you". My basic needs will be put aside until your every perceived need or demand is satisfied.

Hidden contract or agenda: I will do good (be good) if it kills me. I will benefit eventually when you see how valuable I am and decide to value me (be good to/look out for) in return. i.e. - it's up to you to stop me from being killed by my pattern of over-responsible, which is in my outlook perceived as a dynamic of you killing me by you not being more responsible.

Martyr Personality development: aspects of failed individuation with parentification Family history of chronic abuse and domestic violence promote the parentification of the child as a survival strategy, and it is then applied to other relationships as the dominant mode of coping with stress or challenges.

The co-dependent needs to learn boundaries, balance and repose. Silence, lower activity level and time alone or in nature are particularly helpful. You can't give what you don't have. Learn self nourishing techniques so that you have something to give. Co-dependance manifests as dehydration inside the cells causing atrophy, sclerosis and impaired function. The co-dependent manifests cancer, osteoarthritis (over use/ abuse)chronic fatigue and adrenal failure.

Hysteric

Over reaction to every thing as a pre-emptive defense strategy. I am too sensitive or too overwhelmed to handle anything so you (he, she, it) have to change.

Hidden contract or agenda: I cannot protect myself. I am a good person who is a victim of the bad dangerous world through no fault of my own and you have to protect me and fix it and make it okay.

Personality development: walking wounded

History of violence, incest, torture, rape, war, and any form of Post Traumatic Shock produce this defense system. The hysteric looks for 'affirmative action' as a solution in order to redress past or historic wrong which was probably committed by someone else - not you. This manifests as feeling one has to be given the advantage over you (all or some others) to set things right. It is called feeling entitled. It contains the premise that you must cover part of my share, help me or carry my burden to make up for it, make it fair, make it right. Which is of course, impossible, thus the hysteria.

The hysteric needs to learn to be in the now where the trauma is no longer ongoing. Hysteria manifests physiologically as dehydration both inside the cell and outside the cell escalating the crisis dramatically. They are prone to manifest their defensive styles as stroke, asthma, allergies and MS, among others.

"Heaven will be inherited by every man who has heaven in his soul."

Confucius

DEVELOPING INTUITION

To examine intuition as a function, it can be helpful to break it up into component parts. The five aspects of intuition that I consider most important are Love, Sincerity, Simplicity, Detachment, and Interest.

Love

Love is the vibratory rate or frequency for attunement to a being, because love is the essential nature of every being. Love is the life of the soul. "When one loves, one abstains from judging". (Pir Vilayat Inayat Khan, Alchemical Wisdom Cards) also, when one loves one loses consciousness of self, as one is absorbed in the beloved. Love doesn't consider people's limitations, the way we define them or they define themselves, their race, handicaps, sex, personality, etc.

To love, these things are not real. The kind of love I am referring to is a soul-to-soul relationship. You recognize their perfection, the gloriousness of their being, and you have no inhibitions about loving them unreservedly; but it is not romantic love. That is not an aspect of it. Their soul is an angel and it is the most natural thing to love that angel. This kind of love allows one to overlook the 'clues' that trigger your judgment and effectively block intuition. Your powers of discrimination are important, but when you want to be intuitive, overlook the clues, for they may lead you to believe that something is what it is not.

Sincerity

The depth of your sincerity will determine the depth from which you will access guidance from within. If your need for guidance comes from the depth of your being and you are looking for the purpose of your life or a remembrance of who you are, then you get more intuitive answers. You can develop the depth of your sincerity and keep it from being a game, keep it from being entertainment. Value it. This gives you more clarity.

Simplicity

Accept your messages in their simplest form and use them. Intuition comes in a symbolic language or it comes as a feeling, often very subtle. The more details you require, the more potential for distortion comes into your messages. As our capacity grows, then our understanding grows too, and maybe there will be some detail, but our most powerful inner guidance is usually characterized by utter simplicity.

Detachment

If you seek intuitive guidance and yet are holding on to some limitations as to what will be acceptable as an answer, "anything but... just don't let it be...". If you are protecting that area with your denial, not fully open to Truth in that area, then your intuition will be distorted by your own requirements. If you feel that some answers are more acceptable than others, and some answers are completely unacceptable, then your judgment about these things will stand in the way of your intuition. The quality of openness of heart and mind, a degree of detachment from your own judgments, will help you access the truth.

Interest

Interest helps to focus and hold ones attention for a long time. If you lose interest, you will not get intuitive messages beyond that point. If you are trying to get intuitive messages about something you are not deeply interested in, you will not get very much. Your level of interest has a powerful effect on the depth and quality of your guidance. It is very important that you not underestimate the significance of interest in relationship to your intuition. One of the problems that people face in developing their intuition is that they are not sincerely taking an interest in themselves, because to do this means taking a greater responsibility.

What Supports Intuition

Silence	Prayer, Invocation, Faith (belief)	Spiritual Practice
Balance	Intention	Meditation
Love	Integrity	Spiritual Retreats
Interest	Purity, fasting	Harmony
Great Need	Naturalness, simplicity	Peace

What Blocks Intuition

Resentment

Anger

Confusion

Doubt

Self Pity

Guilt

Motive - manipulation or power over

Exhaustion

Stress, overwhelm

Dehydration

Toxic burden, alcohol, drugs

What Distorts Intuition

Avoidance

Denial

Fantasy

Imagination

Embellishing with details

Prejudice

Attachment

Expectations

Fear

Control issues

Interpretation

Critical

Judgmental outlook - knowledge without love

CONCENTRATIONS FOR FOCUS OF ATTUNEMENTS

Identity, Self Image, Adaptive Self and false ego, overcoming limited self-concept
Health, challenges and healing insights and solutions
Psychology, defenses of the ego, fear, depression, emotional challenges
Spiritual development and practice, soul purpose and calling
Relationships, friend, business, sexual, intimate emotionally, spouse, child, parent
Business, finance and career
History, childhood, family history, past lives
Aura Reading - guidance from awareness of the subtle energy bodies
Masters, Saints, Prophets, Guides and Angels
Locations - home, city, country, planet, solar system, galaxy
Elements - earth, fire, water, air, ether
Objects including crystals and plants
Animals
Politics, social activism
Science, quantum physics and metaphysics
What constitutes enlightenment?
God - source and goal, creator and sustainer of all that is, was or will be
Being and Nonbeing
Shadow as Evil, SATAN -seeing all things as negative (critical/judgement) and
LUCIFERIAN - critical of God. Overcoming the critical outlook
Life, death and the meaning of immortality
Happiness as a form of spiritual guidance

"By the divine power of Almighty God My nerves are healed
My mind is still My heart is at rest My Spirit in Peace Peace, Peace, Peace"

Amen
Inayat khan

PERSONAL SPIRITUAL RETREATS

Retreat work means taking time out of our lives to explore and develop our experience of the inner life. Changing the identity and self concept are more readily accomplished when one makes a shift in priorities from outer to inner, and from urgent to important. A retreat is a conscious process of dismantling the self concept and removing the scaffolding that supports it so that you can be completely free to choose again and be deeply inspired to do so in a way that is meaningful to you. It's about stepping back from the everyday life of nonstop busyness, of schedules, of expectations, and allowing one's focus to shift to inner realities and experiences that we can become present to when we stop participating in all the distractions. A retreat is a rehearsal for the next grandest version of you, the new self image that one is cultivating as the centerpiece of one's life.

The primary retreat practice is silence; doing nothing except being silent. Silence supports not being so easily drawn into a mundane outlook. Silence puts us in touch with something much vaster than our usual perception, and it allows us to more clearly perceive that which is within by shielding the doors of perception from the distractions of worldly illusions. The soul communicates in silence.

The length of time or duration of a personal retreat as well as the focus and intent of the retreat must be chosen carefully to fit the individual circumstances and need. Most healers need mini-retreats of a 1/2 day or a full day at least a couple of times a year as well as a longer retreat of several days to support deeper work of healing or transformation. Mini retreats can be self guided.

Longer retreats are best supported by an experienced retreat guide to ensure coming out of the breakdown process and averting it to a breakthrough of spiritual insight, awakening, realization or of healing and resurrection. End the retreat on a positive note of optimism, joy, enthusiasm and ecstasy. After transformative experiences in retreat work, let those who are important to you know that you are not who you were and who you are now and are becoming so that they can uphold your new identity instead of inadvertently holding you to what you were. Make the changes adamant.

RECOMMENDED PRACTICES FOR SPIRITUAL RETREATS:

Silence
Invocation
Attunement to the Masters, Saints and prophets
Prayer
Meditation
Breath Practices
Light Practices
Shamanic Journeying
Self examination of the subtle bodies
Aura imaging
Vision boards
Music and singing
Sound healing, drums, bowls, bells, flute, strings and keyboard
Poetry
Journaling
Life Review
5 year plan
Ceremony and ritual Mikva - ritual purification, bath with oils, flowers, salts
Chi Gong and free form
Tai Chi
Yoga
Walking Meditation
Nature Walks
Star Gazing
Fasting or light pure diet of broth, tea, fruit and nuts. Longer retreats require heartier fare, maybe lentils and oats

Avoid:

Television
Radio
Newspaper
Magazines
Telephone
Computer
Heavy food and alcohol
Conversation

"Loneliness is today's biggest disease."

Mother Teresa

When people would ask Mother Teresa what they could do, she guided them to first help someone in their own family and next to help one of their neighbors.

PRIMARY ROADBLOCKS TO SELF-REALIZATION AND TRUE SELF-ESTEEM

We don't meditate on bliss to get to bliss. We meditate on ourselves to get to bliss. We meditate on the possibilities and watch them unfurl in the inner life, stimulated by the attention of our concentration, of our energy watching every aspect of itself. Immerse the self in the ancient tradition of self observation and create realization now.

Guilt

This experience is claimed by both the Emotional Body and Moral Body. Guilt arises when fear causes acts of selfishness, dishonesty, greed, trying to get an advantage, being unfair about getting what you want - due to fear of not getting what you want if you are completely authentic and above board. Have we made noble choices? Are we capable of making more noble choices in the future than we were previously? Do we continue to do things that we personally disapprove of? This is one of the ways to create negative karma. A dark night of the heart.

Authenticity means being real, honest, true, and whole, as in integrity, rather than compartmentalized, phony and shallowly convenient. Authenticity develops more profoundly when one accepts that they themselves are the person they have been looking for that is so ideal that they want to live with them forever. Be that person that you would want to live with forever because that is exactly what's happening. That is what's real, and everything else is just a veil over that self. The Self is witnessing in every moment who you choose to be through your response to life's challenges and opportunities. Nothing is truly hidden - all is seen.

The qualities to highlight in your being which overcome guilt are Integrity, Authenticity, Valor and Nobility. Each of us has in the depth of our being an undefilable innocence.
In order to examine one's conscience without defenses, one needs to choose another defender - one who has the necessary qualities of strength, mercy, love, insight, power, wisdom, etc... (Archangel Michael, Christ, a patron saint) so that you no longer have to defend yourself. Pick and invoke a

great being who can defend you better than you can defend yourself and then get on with what you need to be looking at, dealing with and changing in your outlook, in yourself concept.

Archetypes and sentences for use in mastering the experience of guilt:

Krishna and Arjuna - ...If I drive your chariot, can you do this thing that is before you in innocence, confidence and faith?

Christ - Go and sin no more.

Yogananda - Stand immaculate in the light of your conscience.

Pir Vilayat - When one can honestly say, I would not now do what I did then, innocence and honor is restored. "Even though you've broken your vows 10,000 times, come, come again."

Resentment

This experience is claimed by both the Mental Body and Moral Body. Resentment is often justified by being called a keen sense of injustice. Mastering resentment is based on overcoming the sense of entitlement to have things the way you believe they should be. It's about meeting life on its own terms with the inner strength, confidence and resilience to resist criticizing and judging what is wrong and whose fault it is when things don't go as expected or desired. This means overcoming the critical outlook, the belief that you are capable of judging right and wrong, good and bad, based on the evidence as you perceive it. To see where the false ego is really getting one over on you... ask yourself what you are proud to hate. Resentment is a dark night of the mind that obscures one's point of view and reduces insight.

You do not have to be the stick that God beats someone with. You can decline every time. Someone else will always readily pick up the stick. This means refusing to judge others as wrong because limited beings can't get it wrong. There is a department of getting all things right, and that aspect of Divine perfection was never put into the hands of limited beings. It means choosing to overlook that which would trigger your judgement and step back from it, disavow it any true meaningfulness - because that is who you choose to be and not because of anyone else's choices or actions. Make it about who you are and not about who someone else should be or could be.

Forgiveness comes from our own self image, who one conceives oneself to be, more than it comes from one's sense of justice or outlook towards the forgiven. Pain and hurt are ways that the ego defines itself, and to blame that on another as 'I was hurt by this person' is the most common psychological defense of the ego. It is a distancing of ourselves from responsibility and power as well as from pain and vulnerability. The spiritual objective is to reconcile with the irreconcilable. Make peace with your experience. Do not honor pains and slights any more highly than is necessary to make a change in yourself and your circumstances. Choose to see these experiences not as wrong but as valued lessons that make you stronger and wiser - if you are willing.

The qualities to highlight in your being which overcome resentment are Mercy, Compassion, Tolerance, and Forgiveness. This work also takes resilience, strength, courage, and faith so if you're feeling blocked, check to see if you need to clear self-pity first.

Archetypes and sentences for use in mastering the experience of resentment:
Christ - Be of good cheer. Give them your cloak also. Neither do I condemn you.
Job - Where were you when I set the foundations of the heavens? Refuse to judge.
Shiva - transformed every experience through his own intention and the transformation chamber of the heart - drinking poison to save the Universe, negative becomes positive through us.
Pir Vilayat - any knowledge you have of a person without love, is judgement. Never criticize anybody. Step back from your judgements when they arise and disavow them.

Self-Pity

This experience is claimed by both the Soul and Moral Body.
Self pity is an experience that only happens in the dimensions of time and limitation. It does not exist in the eternal. It is about all the things that you don't have, that have been denied to you, or taken from you. It is the experience of separation, grief and loss. The soul is shorn of its wings, of its great powers, of its irrepressible spirit and experiences pain, suffering and limitation; a dark night of the soul. You will need to reorient on the experience if you intend to align with and fulfill its potential, its purpose.

This means highlighting different aspects of your story than you have been, such that you improve your story to the point that the crucifixion on earth becomes a coronation in heaven. Find the beauty in your story and if the beauty is lacking, create beautiful thoughts and interpretations composed of luminous, transcendent ideas, and add them to your story until you create the most perfectly wonderful story that you can. That is your privilege. It is also 70% of your happiness.

The qualities to highlight in your being which overcome self pity are Faith, Strength, Resilience, Confidence, Courage, and Irrepressible Spirit, Self-resurrecting.
    Archetypes and sentences for use in mastering the experience of self pity:
Issiah - I will comfort you as a mother comforts her child.
Baha'u'llah - Nothing can ever happen save that which benefits thee.
Christ -My burden is Light.
Pir Vilayat - Each one experiences his share of the birth pangs of the Universe. It is a privilege. Die before death and resurrect now.
Hazrat Inayat Khan - No person will have an experience that is not meant for them.

With a connection to Source and an exemplar or ideal to follow, you can fully master all three of these challenges or tests as they inform you as to the true nature of being. Breath and heartbeat are a connection to Source. The intelligence of the body can do more than 100,000 things right simultaneously. That is the intelligence that runs the Universe. Exemplars are many and include all the masters, saints and prophets of all times, known and unknown. The ideal is your own contribution and your process of discovering your values, what you are willing to sacrifice for and suffer for and respond from the depth of your being - it's no sacrifice at all. That is the point where your ideals and your values meet, the home of your soul.

These spiritual challenges are in the realm of emotion and feelings and can be hard to change. One says 'I cannot help it. That is just how I feel.' Until you don't. Okay, so feelings do change, but what is it that changes them? Insight, new perspective and changed values - all together these create an updated, improved version of your story and your self concept. How do we get these things? Time provides these things for everybody, even the unconscious. If one seeks to participate in the process consciously it begins with opening the heart, being present and paying attention, and really listening to the deepest heart.

How does one open the heart? The process begins with the intention to do so and progresses only so far as you can go without defenses (like an innocent child) and only so far as you can go without resistance (so relax). One follows the breath and the heartbeat into the inner stillness and stays present with patience to the still small voice within and all its nuances.

Hazrat Inayat Khan said "Pain is the price of the opening of the heart." So, the essence then of spiritual mastery is to not object to the pain. Gurdgeiff referred to this in his discourse on the spiritual practice intentional suffering. The experience of pain is mastered by making it hurt much less - 70% less, because there is no psychological pain. When people will not give up psychological pain they become mentally ill, beginning with the dark nights. We all have them. It's instrumental in our growth. Kierkegaard said, "The sufferer must help himself." How? Be still and know.

To meditate on the heartbeat you can hold a pulse point or you can hold your breath. Either way will bring up conscious awareness of the heartbeat. If holding the breath is difficult, it can be done gradually, holding the breath a shorter amount of time for a longer number of breaths. Put a sacred word, thought or name of God on the breath throughout this practice to focus your intention on your connection to source. Om works well. Kyrie Eleison works well for matters of forgiveness.

"Live life as if everything is rigged in your favor."

Rumi

FULFILLMENT

Fulfillment is every moment of our lives in which we accommodate a perception of perfection. Each moment of appreciation for the perfection in which we live and move and have our being is the fulfillment of the purpose of that moment. The perfection we esteem in a flower, in a crystal, in a companion, or in a shooting star, all these moments of perfection are the fulfillment of the purpose of life. God created the entire Universe just for the possibility of you and what you might do with the perfection that is in you, creating you and sustaining you. You are the fulfillment of the divine purpose in every moment because God is experiencing the perfection of love, harmony and beauty in you by creating you.

Every breath that you take is fulfillment of the indwelling nature to expand and to contract, to rise and to fall, to empty and to fill, a perfect balance through reconciliation of opposites into harmony.

Every thought that you think is fulfillment of your purpose as an extension of the Divine Mind, composing infinite possibilities of engaging you with beauty and reveling in your brilliance when your thoughts are filled with light.

Every impulse that you control is a fulfillment of the self mastery you were created for... and every action that you take is a fulfillment of the Divine Intention that you be an instrument of the unfurling of the purpose and perfection of the Universe, the only being. From the moment of the first burst of light emerging out of darkness, fulfillment is all there ever was or will be. Be still and know fulfillment now.

BE AN ACTIVIST

Get on your soap box. In a world where it seems like nothing matters, it is important to be clear about what is important to you. Know what you care about. Don't fritter your energy away fighting against everything that is wrong. Conserve your energy. Pick your cause and take your stand where it matters most to you. Fight for something. It is more powerful and more empowering than fighting against something.

Come from the heart. Be real about the challenges. Be creative about solutions and apply yourself. Fight for the planet. Work for humanity. Work for all non-human species, for healthy oceans, for dolphins and whales, for safe drinking water. Take an adamant stand for safe food or for safe medicine. Fight for a local park or to save the redwoods. Be sincere and be very well informed. Be involved and be irrepressible for what you believe in with your whole heart.

Much good is done in the world by individuals who are deeply moved in their heart to create positive change. The world stands in awe today at the courageous spirit of Julia Butterfly. In the depth of her being she had clear knowing of what is worth living for and what is worth dying for, so she climbed a tree. She didn't pick up a gun and shoot people. She didn't spend millions to economically enforce her will. She did what one person could do, with the help of a few friends. She climbed a tree and did not come down until the world heard her message. She made a difference in the lives of millions whose hearts responded to her message.

So get out there and do your thing. Speak up about what matters. March for peace or for human rights. Send money, write letters, and show up in person for all those things that really matter to you. Those things that you give yourself to in this way are your real values. The difference between values and ideals is that ideals are what we think we want, but values are what we willingly sacrifice for and pay the price without regard for cost because it comes from our sense of doing what it is that we are here for, fulfilling our deepest purpose.

What is the purpose of life (or the purpose of my life)? It seems there may be more than just one, from our perspective. There is the purpose of glory, for instance. Everything you do, no matter what, glorifies the creator just by the fact that you exist. So, beyond that simple glorification that takes place between created and creator, what other purpose?

My spiritual teacher and world wide spiritual teacher to tens of thousands, Pir Vilayat Inayat Khan, used to say that the Universe is responsive to our input. We are a feedback system, holding a seemingly remote outpost at the furthest edge of creation as we know it and saying back to the Universe what does and does not work, from our perspective, from the perspective of the outpost we have been given to hold. The Universe cares. That is a very bold statement. It means both that the universe is conscious and that it experiences emotion. The universe wants to know what you care about, what matters to you from the perspective the universe has put you in.

What is your contribution? Can I prove that the universe wants this? Not exactly, but there is precedent for this outlook in the scripture called the Apocalypse, considered to be the revelations of spiritual mysticism.

In it, God says to man, "if you are neither hot nor cold, I will spew thee out of my mouth." God wants you to have a preference and to know your preference - without demanding that you should have it. Then there is the privilege of applying the purpose of the life that is given to you, to accomplish good according to your own understanding. If you say you don't know what you want, then you cannot co-operate with the universe in creating that which you want. Is it ungracious of us to say we do not know what we want in the face of apparently infinite options?

It is the heart that knows both our preference and purpose. It is the heart that knows our calling and which cause will put us on our soap box to give expression to our deepest self. Instead of responding to the push of the world by striking out blindly in all directions against what appears to be wrong, we need only to be still and know, to turn within and focus. And then be real about what matters to us and be more present to it and what it seems to require of us. An activist on her soap box is not selling snake oil. She is responding to the deepest call of her life's purpose and doing the very thing for which she was created. The entire universe is continually being created just for the possibility of you and what you might do.

> **"The infinite cherishes the finite, the ephemeral longs for the Eternal, and love never rests."**
>
> **Pir Zia Inayat Khan**

HEALTHY ENVIRONMENT

Lack of sufficient clean water for drinking and hygiene is known to cause at least two million child deaths each year. Water use has grown twice as fast as population over the last century. Industry uses 22%, irrigation 70% and 8% is used by households. One billion people each day do not have access to safe water.

The frogs, newts and toads that are being decimated by infectious water borne fungal disease are going to produce consequences in other parts of the ecosystem as well. The resultant lack of natural predators is scientifically predicted to cause significant increase in some insect populations. That nature's water supply is now unhealthy to amphibians and the natural habitats altered state promotes this fungal disease, which is lethal to frogs, is the current scientific assessment. What to do about it remains in question. Development of anti-fungal treatment is being discussed; however, anything less than restoring healthy, pure, safe water cannot solve this problem.
Upsetting the balance of species among insect pollinators will affect the food chain and it will be responded to by further increased use of chemicals.

Another aspect of collapse of the water based ecosystem is represented by the expanding coastal dead zones where the chemical run off meets the ozone warmed water and creates a state of hypoxia and suffocation of all multicellular life, both plant and animal. Ocean acidification and chemicalization, together with rising ocean water temperatures, is accelerating the threat of mass extinction for many species of sea life, from coral reefs to the oyster beds, and possibly more than three quarters of the species that have been relied upon for human food supplies. This loss of biodiversity of ocean life will no doubt become a promoter of loss of biodiversity among all non-ocean species who have had an ocean dependent food supply. This mass failure of earth's water based ecosystem is mirrored by the simultaneous failure of the internal water ecology of the human body in modern times. The body's water supply and the planet's water supply are the same water. That water is the first priority we need to solve in order to create sustainable health for the planet and for the future of all life on it.

EXPERIENCES IN BECOMING A MEDICAL INTUITIVE

by Cyndy Clapp

I was always jealous of intuitives, especially medical intuitives. How were they able to do that? Who or what were they connecting to be able to access the information? Mentally, intellectually, it made so much sense to me, if you realize that everything on this planet is comprised of bundles of different shapes and sizes of energy. Energy can be proven, can be felt, seen, and recorded; you can't get rid of energy, it just changes shape. So, I believed the concept of being able to access other vibrational planes of energy. But why couldn't I do it? Why couldn't I access that information from wherever it was being stored? Why couldn't I "read "someone? I had witnessed many weird, wack-a-doodle type people who, to my dismay, were not only intuitive, but very accurate in their intuition.

That didn't seem fair. I was a normal, intelligent human being, why couldn't I do it? I realized I couldn't seem to turn my mind off; my mind ruled. My mind judged and criticized and doubted much of any information I received. I met Fravarti and witnessed her incredibly accurate intuitive guidance. No fireworks, bright colors, trumpets blaring announcing her intuitive abilities. She had a calm yet strong trust for the guidance she received. She did not appear to judge the information she received. That is what I wanted to be able to do. I had taken classes in animal communication to learn how to communicate with animals and found out that I was already communicating with animals! Something that came so easily and naturally to me on a daily basis was something that everyone did, I thought. Apparently not. I did not realize that that was intuition. I realized that we are all born with intuitive abilities; it is like a muscle, it gets stronger with more focus, attention and practice. But I still couldn't do it the way that Fravarti did. I wanted to be able to get accurate information to help people, guide them accurately, be of service to humanity, use it to help myself.

The 7 years that I commuted to another city for my job and spent 3 hours in traffic daily, I discovered the ability to become an intuitive commuter. I began to "see" the energy vortices and patterns on the road, and feel the energies around the cars which allowed me the ability to avoid traffic jams and back-ups. Cool, I thought. I was then able to drive more efficiently and shorten my commute time. That was using intuition. But why can't I do that with people –like Fravarti?

I did notice that my intuition was strong in areas where I had an interest. I loved animals, felt a real kinship, brotherhood with them and was interested in them. I was interested in traffic that was frustrating me on a daily basis. I wanted to know why it took me so long to travel 15 miles! I love the human body. I love the mechanics behind this amazing machine that is our bodies. Why couldn't I get clear intuition though? I was continuing my training under Fravarti in my own personal work, becoming more familiar with who I was and who I wasn't.

In my childhood, I had learned to become numb, not to feel, because it was too painful at times to feel. When I did allow myself to feel, I usually felt much anxiety, overwhelm, and over stimulated, chaos. My mind judged that there must be something wrong with me. There is nothing "wrong" with me, it is my body levels being flooded with other people's energies. I WAS intuitive, reading people's energies, I just had not learned how to channel all that I was receiving and, most importantly, I did not know *who I was*. I couldn't differentiate if what I was feeling and intuiting was mine or someone else's energy. I thought that intuition came through my mind.

I have now learned how to filter and distinguish what is someone else's energy and which is mine. Once I could do that, I learned how to hold the image of someone's energy and think about a particular homeopathic remedy or supplement, and know if it felt compatible to them or not. Does it feel like a match to that person? It's like hearing but not using your ears. Sometimes it's more of a feeling. I found that my biggest challenge was my mind, my mental body. It wanted to be either right or wrong and wanted facts to back up the answer or information I was getting.

Well, I don't know everything. I believe that there is an Intelligence in this universe that knows a whole lot more than me! I decided to let myself off the hook. I relaxed and shifted my focus to trying to be a clear channel to receive information rather than thinking I had to learn everything about everything to "know" all the answers and fix people. Whew, what a relief that was! Intuition is not based on fact, it is based on Trust and Faith. No one is getting anything wrong, there are no mistakes. Everyone is having exactly the kind of experience they need at that time to learn whatever it is that they are supposed to learn.

Once I learned to let go of the judgment and criticism, my intuition became stronger. Once I became healthier, mentally, emotionally and physically, my intuition became stronger. I engaged in a dance with cancer for about 5 – 6 years which will clearly give you opportunities to cut through your denials and get really clear about who you really are. Through diet, I have maintained a level of hydration in my physical body so that my faculties are not muddied by toxic build up in my body. Keeping my body's pH at a healthy level has reduced the anxiety, stress and doubt that was blocking me from clarity. There are days when I am simply not real clear, when I am "off my game". I admit to that. I am a beautifully, imperfect, perfect human being. I now consider it an honor to have been given the gift of intuition, and am filled with gratitude for such a system of guidance in my life.

So, am I now able to "do what Fravarti "does? Yes, because of her unwavering love, guidance and belief in me which led me to love and believe in myself. Yes. Because I have studied and interned under her for over 20 years sharing hundreds of cases to be examined by her, corrected by her, by learning breath work, how to do attunements, learning self regulation and control of reactions, by understanding what constitutes sustainable health in the human and animal body, by being witness to her own dances with cancer, asthma and many other maladies that surely would have ended the life of anyone else. I am not Fravarti, but I am Cyndy Clapp, Medical Intuitive. Some days are better than others. I strive for accuracy just as she does. I really look forward to the connection I feel when I tap into my intuition now. I am not so much focused on the answer as I appreciate the opportunity of the process itself. Connecting with the The One, The Creator, the Angels, Guides (physical and non physical, human and animal), the Prophets, all the beings and energies which help to give me clarity and guidance in all areas of my life, personal and professional, is something that I treasure and enjoy. And I honor those abilities I have been given by using them for the good of service to myself and others during my lifetime.

Namaste ~~ Cyndy

APPENDIX A

For medical intuitives in training as well as those in practice, it can sometimes be very practical to have comprehensive lists that highlight most things that would be important to consider. The lists in this appendix have served to create focus points for deeper attunement or further research as needed. The lists promote efficiency when used to narrow ones search in this way. However, sticking to any lists would be rather limiting because there will always be thousands of relevant details that are not conveyed in the actual words on the list. Intuition needs to be free to work outside the constraints of any lists as well as be enhanced by the specific focus suggested by reference to these lists. The list is to help one be thorough, and yet one must always be more thorough still, and seek beyond the range and scope of any list.

As a medical intuitive, I don't receive comprehensive answers about things that I know very little about. Constant study, both of human physiology and of available therapies, helps me be a better channel for clear, concise, effective answers and solutions.

Consistently, nationwide, among the professionals for whom I consult, I have found their greatest limitation to be their lack of knowledge of physiological function from macro to micro. The explanation for why to use the answers provided through my intuitive readings always is due to some specific element of normal physiology to be supported or restored.

"The work of a medical intuitive is not so much the work of a healer as it is the work of a guide. I do not heal people. I share what I have learned about what supports health and healing. The healing that takes place is an expression of the relationship between the patient and the divine physician."

Fravarti

HEALTH CHECKLISTS

Blood Chemistry

Formed elements: Neutrophils, eosinophils (check for parasites when elevated), basophils, lymphocytes (T4 - T8), thrombocytes (check for drug toxicity when elevated), coagulation factors, erythrocytes (red cells), hemoglobin, hematocrit.

Elements

Calcium, chromium, copper, iodine, iron, magnesium, manganese, phosphorus, potassium, selenium, silica, sodium, sulphur, zinc, CoQ10
Brain Levels: serotonin, melatonin, phenylalanine, glutamine, glycine, tryptophan

Thyroid

TSH levels, T4 (given as synthroid or thyroxin), Armour thyroid has both T4 and T3 T3 thyronine - body converts from T4, parathyroid, iodine, Wilson's Thyroid Px affected by chlorinated and fluoridated water, pesticides, dental mercury and acidosis

Adrenals

Cortisol function (stress) elevated levels speed age related deterioration - use Vitamin C to support adrenal recovery
Androgen function (sex hormones are reduced when cortisol is high) Aldosterone function (sodium / fluid balance) - use MSM
Kidneys urine pH (5.1 thru 5.5 is acidosis) ideal is above 6.5 up to 6.8 - use lemon water

Digestive System

Acidophilus - lactobaccillis, bifidis, reuteri, mixed, kyodophilus, babydophilis
Pepsin, hydrochloric acid, pancreatin, bile lobe - liver, bile salts - gall bladder, parotid - left and right
Yeast overgrowth, leaky gut, insulin resistance, food allergies
Parasites: liver, spleen, pancreas, upper digestive, small intestines - deuodenum, jujunem, ileum, large intestine - colon, blood

Vitamins

Floradix - Iron and Herbs, Epresat, Floravital, Kinder Love, Calcium, Magnesium
Vitamin A - deficiency usually due to birth control pills or alcohol
B1, B2, B6, B12, Folic Acid
Biotin
Choline
Inositol
Niacin
Pantothenic acid
PABA
Vitamin C, Ester -C, buffered C
Pycnogenols
Quercitin
bioflavonoids
GSE
Vitamin D 3
Vitamin E as pure d-alpha tocopherol or mixed tocopherols

Heavy Metals and Toxins

Aluminum, arsenic, cadmium, copper, fluoride, lead, mercury, silver.
Pesticides - organophosphates (atrazine, crops) and carbomates (Raid, Black Flag) Petroleum distillates, solvents, radiation poisoning, glyphosate, BT.

Allergies

Tobacco, feathers, dander (cat, dog, rabbit), insects (ants, bees, kissing bugs, spiders) pollen, mold, ammonia, formaldehyde, pesticides, nitrites, sodium benzoate, sodium bisulfite

Tick Born Diseases

Lymes, Anaplasmosis, Ehrlichiosis, Tularemia, Rocky Mountain Spotted Fever

Supplements

Colostrum, Detoxamin, Essiac, Elderberry, pycnogenols, omega 3 fish oils, magnesium, zinc, ProGest cream, testoserone gel, MSM, DHEA, melatonin, aloe vera, quercitin, iodine, 5HTP, Calms Forte, Flor-Essence, Masculini-T

Orthomolecular Therapies

L-alanine, L-arganine (impotence), L-asparganine, L-carnitine (acetyl L-carnitine, brain), L-cysteine, NAC - N acetyl cysteine, acetyl choline
GABA gamma amino butric acid (especially for anxiety), L-glutamine (thyroid)
L-glutathione, L-glycine, L-histadine, Inosine, L-isoleucine, L-Lysine (herpes)
L-methionine, L-ornithine, L-phenylalanine, DL-phenylalanine (DLPA)
L-proline, L-serine, phosphytidal serine (HTH), Taurine, L-threonine, tyrosine
L-acetyl tyrosine, L-valine, creatine, vanadyl sulphate, chromium
GLA - gamma linoleic acid (primrose oil or black current), Lecithin, octocosanol (wheatgerm oil), Alpha Lipoic acid, flax oil
Mushrooms - maitake, cordyceps, shiitake, reishi
Wheat grass, chlorella, spirulina, Green Vibrance, Barley Green

Glandulars

Adrenal, lung, lymph/spleen, ovary/uterus, pituitary, pineal, prostate, liver, thyroid, thymus

Botanicals

Ashwaganda, bladderwrack, black walnut, burdock, bupleurum, chapparral, cayenne, clover, cranberry, dandelion, garlic, ginko, goldenseal, ginger, hawthorne, juniper berries, kelp, mistletoe, milk thistle, oregano oil, olive leaf, phytoestrogens, red yeast rice, schizandra, wormwood artemesia, GSE

Cell Salts

1. calc. fluor	4. ferrum phos.	7. kali sulph.	10. nat. phos.	13. biochemic phos.
2. calc. phos.	5. kali mur.	8. mag. phos	11. nat. sulph.	14. Bioplasma
3. calc. sulphate	6. kali phos.	9. nat. mur.	12. silica	

Theraputic Modalities: chiropractic, cranial/sacral, osteopathic, energy work, accupuncture, massage (rolfing, neuromuscular, lymphatic, reflexology),
Chelation and I.V. therapy, castor oil, jin shen
Acupuncture
Acupressure
Apitherapy - Bee venom, for arthritis and MS. Bee pollen, propolis, royal jelly and honey (topically for skin)

Aromatherapy

Diffuser with oils, doTerra CPFG oils, Kaliana spray, Kneipp baths Valerian and Hops, and Lavender, Rosemary

Ayurvedic Medicine

3 doshas: Vata (wind), Pita (fire), Kapha (water)
Panchakarma - 5 step cleansing with herbs, massage, and enemas Pranayama - breathing exercise
Yoga

Bach Flower Remedies

Agrimony, Aspen, Beech, Centaury, Cerato, Cherry Plum, Chestnut Bud, Chicory, Clematis, Crab Apple, Elm, Gentian, Gorse, Heather, Holly, Honeysuckle, Hornbeam, Impatiens, Larch, Mimulus, Mustard, Oak, Olive, Pine, Red Chestnut, Rock Rose, Rock Water, Scleranthus, Star of Bethlehem, Sweet Chestnut, Vervain, Vine, Walnut, Water Violet, White Chestnut, Wild Oat, Wild Rose, Willow, Rescue Remedy

Body Work

Alexander technique - postural, muscle relaxing. Use for posture

Feldenkrais - posture and movement. Use for knee pain and stroke recovery
Rolfing - alignment, release the fascia. Use for trauma recovery
Trager - psychophysical integration. Use for MS
Neuro-muscular massage - trigger point therapy. Includes Bonnie Prudden pain therapy
Chiropractic - arthritis, bursitis, frozen joints
Osteopathic Cranial/Sacral - trauma release, emotional release
Reflexology - blood pressure,lymphatic circulation, kidney support
Lymphatic drainage massage - especially for cancer patients, congestive heart disease
Ear Candling - for wax removal (never use during acute fever or infection)

Chinese Medicine

Restores balance between Yin/Yang, excess vs deficient or stagnant cool/cold, dark, moist, winter vs hot/warm, light dry, summer
5 element system - pungent herbs for the lungs, sour for the liver, sweet for pancreas and spleen, bitter for heart and salts for kidneys.

Hydrotherapies

Kneipp - Hops and Valerian, Lavender and Rosemary. Whirlpool or hot tub therapy
Hot water - relaxes, calm, and stimulates elimination of toxins. Sea salt or epsom salts
Cold water - fever reducer. Cold compresses for inflamed joints, injury or burns
Contrast hot/cold - circulation, congestion, stimulation
Herbal compresses or poultices
Enemas, basti or colonics
Salt baths, salt scrubs, sitz baths, foot baths
Dry brush
Edgar Cayce Caster Oil Pack

Diets

Asian - Soy protein, rice and vegetables
Macrobiotic - sea vegetables, fish - no meat, eggs or refined foods
Mediterranean - olive oil, fish, garlic, red wine, complex carbs
Vegetarian/Vegan - no dairy, meat or eggs
Raw Food diet - healing or cleansing. Gerson Diet and protocols
Fasting or modified fasting
Zone diet - 30% protein, 30% fat, 30% carbs

Blood Type diet (D'Adamo)
Celiac diet - no wheat, spelt, barley or gluten
Candida diet
Paleo diet
Rotation diet or Elimination diet Feingold diet - organic, no additives
Lemon in water or add Celtic salt

Foods And Exclusion Diets

Pork, beef, processed meats, chicken, eggs, dairy, non-organic dairy, soy, corn, wheat, Celiac, barley, rye, Grains (paleo-diet), yeast, peanuts, saccharin, aspartame (Nutrasweet), HFCS, Splenda, sorbitol, MSG, salt, tomatoes, oranges (or juice), coffee, black tea, caffeine, chocolate, margarine, rancid oils, processed foods, sodas, juice, sugar, grapes, berries, wine, alcohol, Nuts - pecan, walnut, cashew, filbert, macadamia eggplant, potatoes, peppers, lima beans, vinegar
Seafood - crab, shellfish, scallops, shrimp, oyster, clam, lobster, tuna, swordfish

Psychotherapy and Body / Mind therapies

Hypnotherapy Meditation
Relaxation techniques, guided imagery - stress, anxiety management
Emotional Freedom Technique - tapping
Prayer Jungian
Cognitive Behavior Therapy
Neuro-linguistic programming
Biofeedback - (depression and Irritable bowel syndrome)

Chelation

Oral - calcium EDTA - 1 to 2 grams, per dose 2 x day for 2 to 3 weeks
I.V. EDTA
I.V. Vitamin C - 25 grams to 50 grams per drip
I.V. ozone
I.V. hydrogen peroxide
I.V. Alpha lipoic acid - 3 cc's to 5 cc's per drip
Glutathione - slow I.V. push 500 mg to 3 grams (increase gradually)
Detoxamin - calcium Disodium EDTA, 750 mg suppositories x 6 weeks
DMSA chelation - 300 mg capsules, 2 per dose 2 x day for 3 to 5 weeks (or I.V.)
DMPS also 600 mgs 2 x day for 3 to 5 weeks (or I.V.)

Zeolite Clay, Bentonite Clay - colon detox, use with Dr. Miller's Holy Tea
Ultraviolet blood irradiation

Hyperbaric Oxygen

Energy Work

Distance healing or laying on of hands
Making water remedies, blessing or charging the water
Reiki
Chi Gong - perception, presence, focus, breathing
Tai Chi - mastery, inner strength, balance
Access Consciousness - bars, identity work, repatterning

Exercise

Aerobic, jumper, bicycle, swimming, hula hoop, stretch and tone, resistance bands, pilates, yoga
walking or interval with skipping, jog or running, skating, martial arts - Taekwondo, Karate, Judo

PREDISPOSITIONS CHECKLIST

Central Nervous System

Bells palsy
Cerebral Palsy
Carbon Monoxide
Parkinson's
Huntington's
Vertigo
ADD & ADHD
MCS or environmental illness
MS

Reproductive System

Dysmenorrhea, PMS
Early menopause, amenorrhea
Estrogen dominance
Endometriosis
Fibroid tumor
Fibrocystic breast
Hysterectomy
Venereal disease, STD's
Vaginal infection, Chlymidia, yeast
Condyloma
HPV, genital warts
Cervical dysplasia
Sterility

Respiratory System

Asthma, allergic or exercise induced
Bronchitis
Pneumonia
Emphysema
COPD
Tuberculosis
Tuberculosis Silicosis/asbestosis

Digestive System

Appendicitis

Pancreatitis

Gastritis

Liver, hepatitis, jaundice

Gallbladder and stones

Colitis, Ileitis, Crohn's

Celiac

Irritable Bowel Syndrome

Leaky Gut Syndrome

Insulin resistance/ syndrome X

Obesity

Acidosis

Malabsorption/malnutrition

PREDISPOSITIONS CHECKLIST

Impotence

Prostate

Pregnancy (also ectopic)

Progesterone, low

Fetal demise or miscarriage

Premature labor, dysfunctional labor

CPD, C- section

Diverticulitis

Candida / yeast overgrowth

Allergies

Headache or migraine

Hernia

Acid reflux

Constipation, hemorrhoids

Urinary System

Bladder, cystitis

Interstitial cystitis

Incontinence, enuresis

Urethral stricture

Kidney stones

Bright's disease

Polycystic kidneys

Renal hypertension

Eczema

Spinal & Bones

Disks, degenerative

Osteoporosis, hips, knees, spine

TB of bones/joints

Bone cysts

Osteomyelitis

Chronic low back syndrome

Arthritis - osteo/rheumatoid

Scoliosis

PREDISPOSITIONS CHECKLIST

1. Acne
2. Adrenals - Addisons, Cushings
3. AIDS or ARC
4. ALS - Amyotrophic lateral sclerosis
5. Alzheimer's and other dementias
6. Anaphylaxis
7. Anemia or sickle cell anemia
8. Aneurism
9. Atherosclerosis, coronary artery disease
10. Arthritis - osteoarthritis
11. Arthritis - rheumatoid
12. Autism
13. Bursitis and intra-patellar bursitis
14. Chemical exposure
15. Chronic fatigue syndrome, Epstein/Barr
16. Cataracts
17. CMV
18. Diabetes
19. Epilepsy
20. Fibromyalgia
21. Fetal alcohol syndrome
22. Glaucoma
23. Heart attack
24. Heart valve or defect, syncope, AVS
25. Heavy metal toxicity
26. Herpes
27. Hypertension
28. Hypoglycemia
29. Lice, crabs or scabies
30. Lupus
31. Leprosy
32. Lyme disease
33. Mononucleosis
34. Morgellon's
35. Multiple Sclerosis
36. Muscular dystrophy
37. Myasthenia gravis
38. Parasites
39. Pesticides
40. Phlebitis, DVT
41. Parkinson's
42. Psoriasis
43. Psoriatic arthritis
44. Radiation
45. Retardation
46. Ring worm, tinea
47. Seborrheic dermatitis
48. Seizures - non-epileptic
49. Shingles
50. Staphyloccus and MRSA
51. Streptococcus
52. Stroke
53. Thyroid - hypo or hyper
54. TMJ
55. Warts
56. Whooping cough
57. Skin cancer

Mental Health

Depression

Manic or Bi-polar disorder

Dementia

Psychosis

Schizophrenia

Anxiety disorder, panic

Organic brain syndrome

Multiple personality

OCD

PTSD

Psychoneurotic disorder

Addiction

Alcoholism and dry drunk

Drugs - prescription and non

Food - bulimia/anorexia

Sex / porn

Co-dependency / love

Compulsive personality

Gambling

Shopping

Religion

Hoarding

TOP PRODUCT RECOMMENDATIONS

Over the years in which she has answered nearly a million questions as a medical intuitive, Fravarti has recommended these excellent products and supportive therapies tens of thousands of times.

CBD Hemp Oil by Prime My Body at Fravarti.com

Clayton Nolte's Deluxe Enhanced Water Structuring Units - for an unlimited amount of structured water at home or traveling. Best price at Fravarti.com

Penta Water - the best therapeutic grade of commercial bottled structured water

Rescue Remedy and other Nelson Bach Remedies including Red Chestnut and Impatiens

Homeopathic Laboratories pharmacy and Treatment Options (txoptions. com)1-800-234-8879 to order your remedies

Similisan Eye Drops, Allergy Eyes

Gaia Herbs including Oil of Oregano and Chinese mushrooms

Sssting Stop by Boericke and Tafel - topical for bug bites including mosquitos, ants

MediNatura - topical support to provide relief for sprains and bruises

Calendula ointment by Hylands as well as their Calms Forte

Vespera Serum by Exuvience - scar removal, skin renewal, precancerous spots. Exuvience is the 4 time winner of the Laureat Award for skin care products and I happily recommend most of their products

Kneipp Aromatherapy baths - 1-800-937-4372 or KneippUS.com

Edgar Cayce Castor Oil Packs

Floradix Liquid Vitamins including: Epresat, Floravital, Kinder Love

Flor-Essence Liquid Detox formula by Flora

Essiac Tea and Powder

Natural Calm by Natural Vitality - Magnesium in an easily assimilated form

Super Quercetin, 1 gram capsules by Bluebonnet - to reduce allergic response

Mega Quercetin by Solaray

Vitamin C, 1 gram capsules by Nature's Way

CoQ10 by Solgar, 400 mgs., for brain and circulation

ProGest Cream by Emerita - topical progesterone cream for hormone balance

Nordic Naturals Complete Omega's

Vitamin E - pure d-alpha tocopherol (not mixed tocopherols) by Country Life
Maca Powder by Indigenous Nutrition.com
Pure Joy Planet.com for raw food cookbooks and videos, nut milk bags, recipes
Essential Enzymes by Source Naturals - digestive and pancreatic support
Udo's Super 8 Probiotics - for upper digestive support
Reuteri by Natures' Way Primadophilis - for colon health, yeast, arsenic and toxins
Babydophilis by Country Life
Dr. Miller's Holy Tea - for digestive healing, available online inc. on Amazon
Vitacost.com - for discount supplements
Beret Jane Miracle Salve, Aromatherapy & Personal Care Products. beretjane.com or 844-888-2100
Kaliana Aromatherapy Mists and Oils - change your mood instantly
Light Therapy Flashlights by LEDwholesalers at Amazon.com"

"My job is to guide people in making the very best choices to support health and healing. If you want the best results, use the best products."

Fravarti

ABBREVIATIONS

5HTP - essential amino acid that raises serotonin
ALA - alpha lipoic acid
ALS - Amyotropic Lateral Sclerosis
BHA - butylated hydroxyanisole
BHT - butylated hydroxytoluene
BPA - biphenyl alanine
BT - bacillus thuringiensis
BVO - bromenated vegetable oil
CF - cystic fibrosis
COPD - congestive, obstructive pulmonary disease
CP - cerebral palsy
CPTG - Certified Pure Therapetic Grade
DHA - docosahexaenoic acid
DMAE - dimethyl amino ethairol, to chelate the brain & support the acetylcholine cycle
DMPS - dimercapto propanesulfonic acid
DMSA - dimercapto succinic acid, remove lead & mercury
EFA's - essential fatty acids
HCG - human chorionic gonadotropin
HCL - salt
HFCS - high fructose corn syrup
GMO - genetically modified organism
GSE - grapefruit seed extract
IUD - intrauterine device
1.U. - international units
1.V. - intravenous
LED - light emitting diode
MCI - myocardial infarction
MCT - hydrochloric acid
MRI - magnetic resonance imaging
MS - multiple sclerosis

MSG - monosodium glutamate
MSM - methylsulfonylmethane
NAC - N-acetyl cysteine
NACL - salt
OTC - over the counter
PABA - para-aminobenzoic acid - a B vitamin
PTSD - post traumatic stress disorder
SOD - super oxydismutase
STD - sexually transmitted disease
TBHQ - tert-Butylhydroquinone

RESOURCES AND SUPPORTIVE MEASURES

Homeopathic Remedies:

TX Options/Homeopathic Labs: 1 (800) 234-8879 www.homeopathiclaboratories.com
    King of Prussia, PA (Professionals: 1 (800) 456-7818)
1800Homeopathy: 1 (800) 466-3672, www.1800homeopathy.com, Richford, VT
    (Standard & Hylands)
Hahnemann Labs: 1 (888) 427-6422, www.hahnemannlabs.com, San Rafael, CA
Homeopathy Overnight: 1 (800) 276-4223, www.homeopathyovernight.net, Cottage Grove, OR
Village Green Apothecary: 1 (800) 869-9159, www.myvillagegreen.com, Bethesda, MD
Remedy Source: 1 (301) 610-6649, http://www.remedysource.com, Bethesda, MD,
    (Washington Homeopathic Products)
Ainsworth: 44 (0) 1883 340 332, http://www.ainsworths.com/London, England

To Purchase Vitamins, Supplements, Topical Aids & Bach Flower Remedies:

Vitacost: http://www.vitacost.com
Vitamin Shoppe: http://www.vitaminshoppe.com
purformulas.com

Books and Educational Resources:

Homeopathy, Beyond Flat Earth Medicine, by Timothy R. Dooley:
    http://www.beyondflatearth.com
Mastering Homeopathy, the Art of Permanent Cure, by Fravarti: http://www.fravarti.com/store
Homeopathic Educational Services: http://www.homeopathic.com
Complementary Medicine Association: http://www. compmed.com
National Center for Homeopathy: http://www.nationalcenterforhomeopathy.org
Eat Right for Your Blood Type, by Peter D'Adamo: http://www.4yourtype.com

Conscious Eating, by Gabriel Cousens, MD: http://www.gabrielcousens.com
Pure Joy Planet, Raw Food Website & Nut Milk Bags: http://www.purejoyplanet.com

Recommended Products Water:

Penta Water http://www.pentawater.com
Clayton's DE water structuring units http://www.fravarti.com/store

Emotional Body Support :

Rescue Remedy and other Nelson Bach Flower Remedies www.bachflower.com
Beret Isaacson, Aromatherapist: www.beretjane.com, beret@beretjane.com,
Kaliana Aromatherapy Mists & Oils: www.kaliana.com
Kneipp Aromatheraphy Baths: http://www.kneippus.com

Probiotics:

Primadophilis Reuteri, by Nature's Way: http://www.naturesway.com/Products/Probiotics/14241-Primadophilus-Reuteri
Udo's Super 8 Probiotics: http://www.udoerasmus.com/products/probiotics_super8
Maxi-Baby Dophilis, by Country Life: http://www.countrylifevitamins.com/product

Digestive Support:

Essential Enzymes, by Source Naturals: http://www.sourcenaturals.com/products
Dr. Miller's Holy Tea: (available at http://www.amazon.com; not available in stores)

Topical Support:

Sssting Stop, by Boericke & Tafel: (available at www.vitacost.com)
Calendula Ointment, by Boiron: (http://www.boironusa.com) or Waleda: (http://usa.weleda.com)
Traumeel Ointment, by Heel: http://www.traumeel.us/
Vespera Serum, by Exuvience: (scar removal, skin renewal; 4x winner of the Laureate Award for skin care products) Available at ULTA or http://www.ariva.com/

Sleep Aids:

Calms Forte, by Hylands: www.hylands.com/products/hylands-calms

Hormonal:

ProGest Cream, by Emrita: http://www.emerita.com
Masculini-T, by Life Seasons: http://www.lifeseasons.com

Physical Body Support:

Edgar Cayce Castor Oil Packs: http://www.edgarcayce.org,
Similisan Eye Drops, Allergy Eyes: http://similasannaturalremedies.com

Miscellaneous Food, Supplements, and Supportive Products:

Agave Nectar, raw/organic, by Madhava: http://www.madhavasweeteners.com/
Codyceps & Reishi Mushrooms, available at: http://www.vitacost.com
Co Q10 Megasorb 400 mg, by Solgar: http://www.solgar.com/SolgarProducts/Megasorb-CoQ-10-400-mg-Softgels.htm
Essiac Powder & Tea: http://www.essiacproducts.com/
Gaia Herbs: http://www.gaiaherbs.com/
Natural Calm Magnesium, by Natural Vitality: http://naturalvitality.com/
Vitamin C 1000 mg Capsules, by Nature's Way: http://www.naturesway.com/products/Immune-System/15464-Vitamin-C-1000- with-Bioflavonoids.aspx
Vitamin E (pure d-alpha tocopheryl, not mixed) 400 mg, by Country Life: http://www.country-life.com/store/natural-vitamin-e-400-iu
Flora Products, Epresat, Flor-Essence, Floradix, Iron & Herbs, Kinder Love, Sambu Guard: http://www.florahealth.com/home_usa.cfm
Oil of Oregano capsules, Gaia Herbs
Sunflower Seed Oil, by Spectrum: http://www.spectrumingredients.com/product/ed_oils/sun_HO_org.html
Super Quercetin, by Blue Bonnet: http://www.bluebonnetnutrition.com/product/98/Super_Quercetin%AE_Vcaps
Maca Powder: http://www.IndigenousNutrition.com

Printed in the United States
By Bookmasters